Handbook of Exercise Testing

Handbook of Exercise Testing

Victor F. Froelicher, M.D.
Professor of Medicine, Division of Cardiovascular Medicine, Stanford University School of Medicine, Stanford; Director, ECG and Exercise Laboratory and Cardiac Rehabilitation, Veterans Affairs Palo Alto Health Care System, Palo Alto, California

Susan Quaglietti, R.N., M.S.N.
Assistant Clinical Professor, School of Nursing, University of California, San Francisco; Adult Nurse Practitioner, Cardiology Division, Veterans Affairs Palo Alto Health Care System, Palo Alto, California

Little, Brown and Company
Boston New York Toronto London

First Edition

Library of Congress Cataloging-in-Publication Data

Froelicher, Victor F.
Handbook of exercise testing / Victor F. Froelicher, Susan Quaglietti.
p. cm.
Includes index.
ISBN 0-316-29429-2
1. Exercise tests—Handbooks, manuals, etc. I. Quaglietti, Susan. II. Title.
[DNLM: 1. Exercise Test—handbooks. WG 39 F926h 1995]
RC683.5.E94F763 1995
616.1'220754—dc20
DNLM/DLC
for Library of Congress 95-21519
CIP

Printed in the United States of America

RRD-VA

Editorial: Nancy Megley and Richard L. Wilcox
Production Services: P. M. Gordon Associates
Cover Designer: Mike Burggren
Flow charts are from V. Froelicher. *EXTRA—The Exercise Testing Reporting Guide.* Menlo Park, CA, 1995.

To our families, who encourage us to learn . . .
To our students, who are eager to learn . . .
To our patients, who allow us to continue to learn.

Contents

IV. Applications of Exercise Testing

Preface

We decided to write the *Handbook of Exercise Testing* essentially for two reasons. First, we were challenged to produce an algorithmic approach to exercise testing. Second, we wanted to make a source of knowledge regarding exercise testing available in a pocket-sized, easy-to-read version for internists, family practitioners, and advanced practice nurses now doing many of the exercise tests previously performed by cardiologists. With this transition in use of the test, an efficient transfer of knowledge must take place. The standard exercise ECG test will remain a valuable and reliable tool only if consistent principles are followed.

We hope that our experience training hundreds of residents and nurse practitioners serves our readers well in this book. It is important that the standard exercise ECG test be performed following established principles so that it is not superseded by the newer modalities of nuclear perfusion and echocardiography. These modalities have not been as thoroughly evaluated as the standard exercise ECG and add useful additional clinical information in only a fraction of patients.

We wanted the handbook to supplement and be consistent with the excellent guidelines released by the AHA/ACC and the ACSM. For this reason we were careful to espouse the following principles:

- The treadmill protocol should be adjusted to the patient since one protocol is not appropriate for all patients.
- Report exercise capacity in METS, not minutes of exercise.
- Hyperventilation prior to testing is not indicated.
- ST measurements should be made at STO (J-junction) and ST depression should be considered abnormal only if horizontal or downsloping.
- When being tested for diagnostic purposes, patients should be placed supine as soon as possible in postexercise, with a cool-down walk avoided in order for the test to have its greatest diagnostic value.
- The ECG at 3-minutes' recovery is critical to include in analysis of the ST response.
- Measurement of systolic blood pressure during exercise is extremely important and exertional hypotension is ominous; with current technology, only manual BP measurement techniques are valid.

- Age-predicted heart rate targets are largely useless because of the wide scatter for any age; a relatively low heart rate can be maximal for a patient of a given age and submaximal for another. Thus, a test should not be considered non-diagnostic if a percentage of age-predicted maximal heart rate (i.e., 85%) is not reached.

The most dangerous circumstances in the exercise testing lab are:

1. Testing patients with aortic valvular disease because they can have cardiovascular collapse (and it is extremely hard to resuscitate them because of the outflow obstruction).
2. When patients exhibit ST segment elevation without diagnostic Q waves (which is due to transmural ischemia). This can be associated with dangerous arrhythmias and infarction; it occurs in about 1 of 1000 clinical tests.
3. When a patient with an ischemic cardiomyopathy exhibits severe chest pain due to ischemia (angina pectoris). In this instance, a cool-down walk is advisable since the ischemia can worsen in recovery.
4. When a patient develops exertional hypotension accompanied by ischemia (angina or ST depression) or when it occurs in a patient with a history of CHF, cardiomyopathy, or recent MI.
5. When a patient with a history of sudden death or collapse during exercise develops PVCs that become frequent. In this instance, a cool-down walk is advisable since the PVCs can increase in recovery.

Appreciation of these circumstances can help you avoid any complications in your exercise lab.

We would like to thank our editor Nancy Megley for help with planning, careful reading of early drafts, and suggestions. Thanks, also, Nancy for putting up with our urgency. Our publishing team, including Richard Wilcox, has been most helpful (thanks to Richard for resizing the VISIO flow diagrams). Thanks also to Stephanie for freeing us from any conflict with prior writing projects. Further thanks to our students, who encouraged us that another exercise testing book was needed.

Good luck to our readers. We hope this handbook enables you to apply this wonderful testing modality to benefit patients. We hope that this knowledge base guides those in the field through the exercise test. Ultimately, it should give you confidence to manage patients with heart disease and help you decide when it is appropriate to refer the patient to a cardiologist.

V.F.F.
S.Q.

Basics

Notice. The indications and dosages of all drugs in this book have been recommended in the medical literature and conform to the practices of the general medical community. The medications described do not necessarily have specific approval by the Food and Drug Administration for use in the diseases and dosages for which they are recommended. The package insert for each drug should be consulted for use and dosage as approved by the FDA. Because standards for usage change, it is advisable to keep abreast of revised recommendations, particularly those concerning new drugs.

Exercise Physiology

Exercise physiology is the study of the physiologic responses and adaptations that occur as a result of acute or chronic exercise. Exercise is the body's most common physiologic stress, and it places major demands on the cardiopulmonary system. For this reason, exercise can be considered the most practical test of cardiac perfusion and function. Exercise testing is a noninvasive tool to evaluate the cardiovascular system's response to exercise under carefully controlled conditions. The adaptations that occur during an exercise test allow the body to increase its resting metabolic rate up to 20 times, during which cardiac output may increase as much as six times. The magnitude of these adjustments is dependent on age, gender, lean and total body mass, type of exercise, fitness, and the presence or absence of heart disease.

ENERGY AND MUSCULAR CONTRACTION

Muscular contraction is a complex mechanism involving the interaction of the contractile proteins actin and myosin in the presence of calcium. Myosin and actin filaments in the muscle slide past one another as the muscle fibers shorten during contraction. The source of energy for this contraction is supplied by adenosine triphosphate (ATP), which is produced in the mitochondria. Adenosine triphosphate is stored as two components, adenosine diphosphate (ADP) and phosphate (Pi), at specific binding sites on the myosin heads.

The sequence of events that occur when a muscle contracts involves calcium and two inhibitory proteins, troponin and tropomyosin. Voluntary muscle contraction begins with the arrival of electrical impulses at the myoneural junction, initiating the release of calcium ions. Calcium is released into the sarcoplasmic reticulum, which surrounds the muscle filaments, binds to a special protein, troponin-C, which is attached to both tropomyosin (another protein that inhibits the binding of actin and myosin) and actin. When calcium binds to troponin-C, the tropomyosin molecule is removed from its blocking position between actin and myosin, the myosin head attaches to actin, and muscular contraction occurs.

Adenosine triphosphate, the main source of energy for muscular contraction, is produced by oxidative phosphorylation. The major fuels for this process are carbohydrates (glycogen and glucose) and free fatty acids. At rest, equal amounts of energy are derived from carbohydrates and fats. Free fatty acids contribute greatly during low levels of exercise, but greater amounts of energy are derived from carbohydrates as exercise progresses. Maximal work relies virtually entirely on carbohydrates. Because endurance performance is directly related to the rate at which carbohydrate stores are depleted, a major advantage exists in having greater glycogen stores in the muscle and in deriving a relatively greater proportion of energy from fat during prolonged exercise.

Oxidative phosphorylation initially involves a series of events that take place in the cytoplasm. Glycogen and glucose are metabolized to pyruvate through glycolysis. If oxygen is available, pyruvate enters the mitochondria from the sarcoplasm and is oxidized to a compound known as acetyl CoA, which then enters a cyclical series of reactions known as the Krebs cycle, the byproducts of which are CO_2 and hydrogen. Electrons from hydrogen enter the electron transport chain, yielding energy for the binding of phosphate (phosphorylation) from ADP to ATP. This process, oxidative phosphorylation, is the greatest source of ATP for muscle contraction. A total of 36 ATP per molecule of glucose are formed in the mitochondria during this process.

The mitochondria can only produce ATP for muscle contraction if oxygen is present. At higher levels of exercise, however, total body oxygen demand may exceed the capacity of the cardiovascular system to deliver oxygen. The term anaerobic (without oxygen) glycolysis has been used to describe the synthesis of ATP from glucose under these circumstances. This term has been replaced with "oxygen independent" glycolysis as "anaerobic" incorrectly implies glycolysis occurs only when there is an inadequate oxygen supply. Under such conditions, glycolysis progresses in the cytoplasm in much the same way as aerobic metabolism until pyruvate is formed. However, electrons released during glycolysis are taken up by pyruvate to form lactate acid. Rapid diffusion of lactate from the cell inhibits any further steps in glycolysis. Thus, oxygen-independent glycolysis is quite inefficient; two ATP per molecule of glucose is the total yield from this process. Lactate contributes to fatigue by increasing ventilation and inhibiting other enzymes of glycolysis. It also serves as an important precursor for liver glycogen during exercise.[1]

MUSCLE FIBER TYPES

The body's muscle fiber types have been classified based on the speed with which they contract, their color, and their mitochondrial content. Type I, or slow twitch fibers, are red and contain high concentrations of mitochondria. Type II, or fast twitch fibers, are white and have small concentrations of mitochondria. Fiber color is related to the degree of myoglobin, which is a protein that both stores oxygen in the muscle and carries oxygen in the blood to the mitochondria. Slow twitch fibers, with their high myoglobin content, are more resistant to fatigue; thus, a muscle with a high percentage of slow twitch fibers is well suited for endurance exercise. However, slow twitch fibers tend to be smaller and produce less overall force than fast twitch fibers. Fast twitch fibers are generally larger and tend to produce more force but fatigue more easily. The speed of contraction for each fiber type is based largely on the activity of an enzyme in the myosin head that combines with ATP.[2]

CARDIOPULMONARY RESPONSE TO ACUTE EXERCISE

Three types of exercise performed by the body can be used to stress the cardiovascular system: isometric, dynamic, and a combination of the two. Isometric exercise, defined as constant muscular contraction without movement (such as hand grip), imposes a disproportionate pressure load on the left ventricle relative to the body's ability to supply oxygen. Dynamic exercise is defined as rhythmic muscular activity resulting in movement and initiates a more appropriate increase in cardiac output and oxygen exchange. In that a delivered workload can be accurately calibrated and the physiologic response easily measured, dynamic exercise is preferred for clinical testing. Using progressive workloads of dynamic exercise, patients with coronary artery disease can be protected from rapidly increasing myocardial oxygen demand. Although bicycling is a dynamic exercise, most individuals perform more work on a treadmill because a greater muscle mass is involved and most subjects are more familiar with walking than cycling.[3]

Dynamic exercise is preferred to isometric exercise for testing because it can be graduated and controlled and puts a volume stress on the heart rather than a pressure stress. However, most activities usually combine both types of exercise in varying degrees.

REFERENCES

1. Brooks GA. The lactate shuttle during exercise and recovery. *Med Sci Sports Exerc* 18:360–368, 1986.
2. Saltin B, Henricksson J, Hugaard E, Andersen P. Fiber types and metabolic potentials of skeletal muscles in sedentary man and endurance runners. *Ann NY Acad Sci* 301:3–29, 1977.
3. Myers J, Buchanan N, Walsh D, Kraemer M, McAuley P, Hamilton-Wessler M, Froelicher VF. Comparison of the ramp versus standard exercise protocols. *J Am Cell Cardiol* 17:1334–1342, 1991.

Specific Responses to Dynamic Exercise

The cardiovascular system responds to acute dynamic exercise with a series of adjustments that ensure (1) active muscles receive blood supply that is appropriate to their metabolic needs, (2) heat generated by the muscles is dissipated, and (3) blood supply to the brain and heart is maintained. This requires a major redistribution of cardiac output along with a number of local metabolic changes.

The usual measure of the capacity of the body to deliver and use oxygen is the maximal oxygen uptake (V_{O_2} max). The limits of the cardiopulmonary system are defined by V_{O_2} max, which can be expressed by the Fick principle:

$$V_{O_2} = \text{cardiac output} \times \text{arteriovenous oxygen difference}$$

Cardiac output must closely match pulmonary ventilation to deliver oxygen to the working muscle. V_{O_2} max is determined by the maximal amount of ventilation (V_E) moving into and out of the lung and the fraction of this ventilation that is extracted by the tissues:

$$V_{O_2} = V_E \times (F_IO_2 - F_EO_2)$$

where V_E is minute ventilation and F_IO_2 and F_EO_2 are the fractional amounts of oxygen in the inspired and expired air, respectively.

The cardiopulmonary limits (V_{O_2} max) are defined by a central component (cardiac output), which describes the capacity of the heart to function as a pump, and peripheral factors (arteriovenous oxygen difference), which describe the capacity of the lung to oxygenate the blood delivered to it and the capacity of the working muscle to extract this oxygen from the blood. Some of the factors that affect cardiac output and arteriovenous oxygen difference are discussed below.

CENTRAL FACTORS

Heart Rate

Sympathetic and parasympathetic nervous systems affect the cardiovascular system's first response to exercise, an increase in heart rate. Sympathetic outflow to the heart and systemic blood vessels increases, while vagal outflow decreases. Of the two major components of cardiac output, heart rate and stroke volume, heart rate is responsible for most of the increase in cardiac output during exercise, particularly at higher levels. Heart rate increases linearly with workload and oxygen uptake. Increases in heart rate occur primarily at the expense of diastolic, rather than systolic time. Thus, at very high heart rates, diastolic time may be so short as to preclude adequate ventricular filling.

The heart rate response to exericse is influenced by several factors including age, type of activity, body position, fitness, the presence of heart disease, medications, blood volume, and environment. Of these, perhaps the most important is age; a decline in maximal heart rate occurs with increasing age.[1] This appears to be due to intrinsic cardiac changes rather than to neural influences. There is a great deal of variability around the regression line between maximal heart rate and age; thus, age-related maximal heart rate is a relatively poor indicator of maximal effort.

Stroke Volume

The product of stroke volume (the volume of blood ejected per heart beat) and heart rate determines cardiac output. Stroke volume is equal to the difference between end-diastolic and end-systolic volumes. Thus, a greater diastolic filling (preload) will increase stroke volume. Alternatively, factors that increase arterial blood pressure will resist ventricular outflow (after load) and result in a reduced stroke volume. During exercise, stroke volume increases to approximately 50% to 60% of maximal capacity, after which increases in cardiac output are due to further increases in heart rate. The extent to which increases in stroke volume during exercise reflect an increase in end-diastolic volume and/or a decrease in end-systolic volume is not entirely clear, but appear to depend on ventricular function, body position, and intensity of exercise.[2-4]

End-Diastolic Volume

In addition to heart rate, end-diastolic volume is determined by two other factors: filling pressure and ventricular compliance.

Filling Pressure

The most important determinant of ventricular filling is venous pressure. The degree of venous pressure is a direct consequence of the amount of venous return. The Frank-

Starling mechanism requires that all of the blood that is returned to the heart will be ejected during systole. As the tissues demand greater oxygen during exercise, venous return increases, which increases end-diastolic fiber length (preload), resulting in a more forceful contraction. Venous pressure increases as exercise intensity increases. Over the course of a few beats, cardiac output will equal venous return.

A number of other factors affect venous pressure and therefore filling pressure during exercise. These include blood volume and the pumping action of the respiratory and skeletal muscles. A greater blood volume increases venous pressure and, therefore, end-diastolic volume by making more blood available to the heart. The intermittent mechanical constriction and relaxation in the skeletal muscles during exercise also enhance venous return. Changes in intrathoracic pressure, which occur with rapid breathing during exercise, facilitate the return of blood to the heart.

Ventricular Compliance

The expandability of the left ventricle is largely determined by structural features of the ventricle. Damage, infiltrative processes or hypertrophy can limit ventricular expandability. Changes most likely are very subtle since the left ventricle causes a sucking pressure as it re-expands after contraction and this negative pressure cannot be easily measured.

End-Systolic Volume

The end result of contraction, the residual or end-systolic volume is dependent on two factors: contractility and afterload.

Contractility describes the forcefulness of the heart's contraction. Increasing contractility reduces end-systolic volume, which results in a greater stroke volume and thus cardiac output. Contractility is quantified by the ejection fraction, the percentage of blood that is ejected from the ventricle during systole. This can be done using radionuclide, echocardiographic, or angiographic techniques but it will be falsely elevated relative to contractility when mitral regurgitation is present.

Afterload is a measure of the force resisting the ejection of blood by the heart. Increased afterload (or aortic pressure, as is observed with chronic hypertension) results in a reduced ejection fraction and increases in end-diastolic and end-systolic volumes. During dynamic exercise, the force resisting ejection in the periphery (total peripheral resistance) is reduced by vasodilation, due to the effect of local metabolites on the skeletal muscle vasculature. Despite a fivefold increase in cardiac output among normal subjects during exercise, mean arterial pressure increases only moderately.

Ventricular Volume Response to Exercise

In normal subjects, the response from upright rest to a moderate level of exercise is an increase in both end-diastolic and end-systolic volumes of 15% and 30%, respectively. As exercise progresses to a higher intensity, end-diastolic volume probably does not increase further, while end-systolic volume decreases progressively. At peak exercise, end-diastolic volume may even decline somewhat, while stroke volume is maintained by a progressively decreasing end-systolic volume.

PERIPHERAL FACTORS (a-V_{O_2} DIFFERENCE)

Oxygen extraction by the tissues during exercise reflects the difference between the oxygen content of the arteries (generally 18 to 20 ml O_2/100 ml at rest) and the oxygen content in the veins (generally 13 to 15 ml O_2/100 ml at rest, yielding a typical a-V_{O_2} difference at rest of 4–5 ml O_2/100 ml—approximately 23% extraction). During exercise, this difference widens as the working tissues extract greater amounts of oxygen; venous oxygen content reaches very low levels, and a-V_{O_2} difference may be as high as 16 to 18 ml O_2/100 ml with exhaustive exercise (exceeding 85% extraction of oxygen from the blood at V_{O_2} max). Some oxygenated blood always returns to the heart, however, as smaller amounts of blood continue to flow through metabolically less active tissues that do not fully extract oxygen. a-V_{O_2} difference is generally considered to widen by a relatively "fixed" amount during exercise, and differences in V_{O_2} max are explained by differences in cardiac output. However, patients with cardiovascular and pulmonary disease exhibit reduced V_{O_2} max values, which can be attributed to a combination of central and peripheral factors.

Determinants of Arterial Oxygen Content

Arterial oxygen content is related to the partial pressure of arterial oxygen, which is determined in the lung by alveolar ventilation and pulmonary diffusion capacity and in the blood by hemoglobin content. In the absence of pulmonary disease, arterial oxygen content and saturation are usually normal throughout exercise, even at very high levels. This is true even among patients with severe coronary disease or chronic heart failure. Patients with pulmonary disease, however, often neither ventilate the alveoli adequately nor diffuse oxygen from the lung into the bloodstream normally. A decrease in arterial oxygen saturation during exercise is another of the hallmarks of this disorder. Arterial hemoglobin content is also usually normal throughout exercise. Naturally, a condition such as anemia would reduce the oxygen carrying capacity of the blood, along with any condition that would shift the O_2 dissociation curve leftward, such as reduced 2,3-diphosphoglycerate, PCO_2, or temperature.

Determinants of Venous Oxygen Content

Venous oxygen content reflects the capacity to extract oxygen from the blood as it flows through the muscle. It is determined by the amount of blood directed to the muscle (regional flow) and capillary density. Muscle blood flow increases in proportion to the increase in work rate and the associated oxygen requirement. The increase in blood flow is brought about not only by the increase in cardiac output, but also by a preferential redistribution of the cardiac output to the exercising muscle. A reduction in local vascular resistance facilitates this greater skeletal muscle flow. In turn, locally produced vasodilatory mechanisms, and possible neurogenic dilatation due to higher sympathetic activity, mediate the greater skeletal muscle blood flow. A marked increase in the number of open capillaries reduces diffusion distances, increases capillary blood volume, and increases mean transit time, thus facilitating oxygen delivery to the muscle.

TYPES OF OXYGEN CONSUMPTION

Two types of oxygen consumption must be considered to understand exercise testing. Total body oxygen uptake and myocardial oxygen uptake are distinct in their determinants and in the way they are measured or estimated. Total body or ventilatory oxygen uptake (VO_2) is the amount of oxygen that is extracted from inspired air as the body performs work. Myocardial oxygen uptake is the amount of oxygen consumed by the heart muscle. Accurate measurement of myocardial oxygen consumption requires the placement of catheters in a coronary artery and the coronary venous sinus to measure oxygen content. Its determinants include intramyocardial wall tension (left ventricular pressure end-diastolic volume), contractility, and heart rate. It has been shown that myocardial oxygen uptake is best estimated by the product of heart rate and systolic blood pressure (double product).[5] This is valuable clinically because exercise-induced angina often occurs at the same myocardial oxygen demand (double product), and thus is one physiologic variable that is useful for evaluating therapy. When this is not the case, the influence of other factors should be suspected, such as a recent meal, abnormal ambient temperature, or coronary artery spasm.

Interaction

Considerable interaction takes place between the exercise test manifestations of abnormalities in myocardial perfusion and myocardial function. The ECG response and angina are closely related to myocardial ischemia (coronary artery disease), whereas exercise capacity, systolic blood pressure, and heart rate responses to exercise are determined by myocardial ischemia, myocardial dysfunction, responses in the periphery, or a combination of the three. Exercise-induced ischemia can cause cardiac dysfunction resulting in exercise impairment and an abnormal systolic blood pressure response, making it difficult to separate the impact of ischemia from the impact of left ventricle dysfunction.

The severity of ischemia or the amount of myocardium in jeopardy is known clinically to be inversely related to the heart rate, blood pressure, and exercise level achieved. However, neither resting nor exercise ejection fraction (nor its change during exercise) correlates well with measured or estimated maximal ventilatory oxygen uptake, even in patients without signs or symptoms of ischemia.[6] Exercise-induced markers of ischemia (angina, ST depression, thallium defects, wall motion abnormalities) do not correlate well with one another.[7] Silent ischemia (i.e., markers of ischemia presenting without angina) does not appear to affect exercise capacity in patients with coronary heart disease. Although cardiac output is generally considered the most important determinant of exercise capacity, the periphery plays an important role in limiting or enhancing exercise capacity.

Myocardial Perfusion

Although heart rate and stroke volume are important determinants of both maximal oxygen uptake and myocardial oxygen consumption, myocardial oxygen consumption has other independent determinants. The relative metabolic loads of the entire body and those of the heart are determined separately and may not change in parallel with a given intervention. Although the heart receives only 4% of cardiac output at rest, it uses 10% of systemic oxygen uptake. The wide arteriovenous oxygen difference across the coronary circulation of 10 to 12 volume percent at rest reflects that oxygen in the blood passing through the coronary circulation is nearly maximally extracted. When the myocardium requires a greater oxygen supply, coronary blood flow must be increased by coronary dilation. During exercise, coronary blood flow can increase through normal coronary arteries up to five times the normal resting flow.

The increased demand for myocardial oxygen consumption required for dynamic exercise is the key to the use of exercise testing as a diagnostic tool for coronary artery disease. Myocardial oxygen consumption cannot be directly measured in a practical manner, but its relative demand can be estimated from its determinants, such as heart rate, wall tension (left ventricular pressure and diastolic volume), contractility, and cardiac work. Although all of these factors increase during exercise, increased heart rate is especially detrimental in patients who have obstructive coronary disease. Increases in heart rate result in a shortening of the diastolic filling period, the time during which coronary blood flow is the greatest. In normal coronary arteries, dilation occurs. In obstructed vessels, however, dilation is limited and flow is decreased by the shortening of the diastolic filling period. This situation results in both inadequate blood flow and oxygen delivery. Changes in this threshold are due to coronary artery spasm.

REFERENCES

1. Hammond HK, Froelicher VF. Normal and abnormal heart rate responses to exercise. *Prog Cardiovasc Dis* 27:271–296, 1985.
2. Plotnick GD, Becker L, Fisher ML, Gerstenblith G, Renlund DG, Fleg JL, Weisfeldt ML, Lakatta EG. Use of the Frank-Starling mechanism during submaxi-

mal versus maximal upright exercise. *Am J Physiol* 251:H1101–H1105, 1986.

3. Ginzton LE, Conant R, Brizendine M, Laks MM. Effect of long-term high intensity aerobic training on left ventricular volume during maximal upright exercise. *J Am Coll Cardiol* 14:364–371, 1989.
4. Higginbotham MB, Morris KG, Williams RS, McHale PA, Coleman RE, Cobb FR. Regulation of stroke volume during submaximal and maximal upright exercise in normal man. *Circ Res* 58:281–291, 1986.
5. Nelson RR, Gobel FL, Jorgensen CR, Wang K, Taylor HL. Hemodynamic predictors of myocardial oxygen consumption during static and dynamic exercise. *Circulation* 50:1179–1189, 1974.
6. McKirnan MD, Sullivan M, Jensen D, et al. Treadmill performance and cardiac function in selected patients with coronary heart disease. *J Am Coll Cardiol* 3:253–261, 1984.
7. Hammond HK, Kelley TL, Froelicher VF. Noninvasive testing in the evaluation of myocardial ischemia: Agreement among tests. *J Am Coll Cardiol* 5:59–69, 1985.

Basics of Applying the Exercise Stress Test

EXERCISE TEST MODALITIES

Numerous modalities have been used to provide dynamic exercise for exercise testing, including steps, escalators, and ladder mills. Today, however, the bicycle ergometer and the treadmill are the most commonly used dynamic exercise devices. The bicycle ergometer is usually cheaper, takes up less space, and makes less noise. Upper body motion is usually reduced, but care must be taken so that isometric exercise is not performed by the arms. The workload administered by the simple bicycle ergometers is not well calibrated and is dependent on pedaling speed. It is too easy for a patient to slow pedaling speed during exercise testing and decrease the administered workload. More expensive, electronically braked bicycle ergometers keep the workload at a specified level over a wide range of pedaling speeds. Treadmills are most commonly used in the United States because Americans are more familiar with walking than bicycling.

EXERCISE PROTOCOLS

The many different exercise protocols in use have caused some confusion regarding how physicians compare tests between patients and serial tests in the same patient. The most common protocols, their stages, and the predicted oxygen cost of each stage are illustrated in Fig. 3-1. When treadmill and bicycle ergometer testing were first introduced into clinical practice, practitioners adopted protocols used by major researchers. The Bruce protocol, which is frequently used for routine clinical testing, uses relatively large and unequal 2- to 3-MET increments in workload every 3 minutes. Because large and uneven workload increments such as these result in a tendency to overestimate exercise capacity, we recommend protocols with smaller and more equal increments. Exercise tests with work increments individualized to yield a duration of approximately 10 minutes are optimal for assessing cardiopulmonary function.[1-3] Among patients with chronic heart failure, small work increments yielding a long test duration result in reduced values for maximal oxygen uptake, minute ventilation, and arterial lactate compared

FUNCTIONAL CLASS	CLINICAL STATUS	O_2 COST ml/kg/min	METS	BICYCLE ERGOMETER	TREADMILL PROTOCOLS															METS
				1 WATT = 6.1 Kpm/min FOR 70 KG BODY WEIGHT Kpm/min	BRUCE 3 MIN STAGES		BALKE-WARE % GRADE AT 3.3 MPH 1 MIN STAGES	USAFSAM		"SLOW" USAFSAM		McHENRY		STANFORD % GRADE AT 3 MPH	STANFORD % GRADE AT 2 MPH	ACIP		CHF		
					MPH	%GR		MPH	%GR	MPH	%GR	MPH	%GR			MPH	%GR	MPH	%GR	
					5.5	20														
					5.0	18														
NORMAL AND I	HEALTHY, DEPENDENT ON AGE, ACTIVITY	56.0	16				26 25 24 23 22 21 20 19 18 17 16 15 14 13 12 11 10 9 8 7 6 5 4 3 2 1													16
		52.5	15					3.3	25							3.4	24.0			15
		49.0	14	1500								3.3	21							14
		45.5	13		4.2	16										3.1	24.0			13
		42.0	12	1350				3.3	20			3.3	18	22.5		3.0	21.0			12
		38.5	11	1200										20.0						11
	SEDENTARY HEALTHY	35.0	10	1050	3.4	14		3.3	15			3.3	15	17.5		3.0	17.5	3.4	14.0	10
		31.5	9							2	25	3.3	12	15.0		3.0	14.0	3.0	15.0	9
		28.0	8	900				3.3	10	2	20			12.5		3.0	10.5	3.0	12.5	8
	LIMITED	24.5	7	750	2.5	12						3.3	9	10.0	17.5			3.0	10.0	7
II	SYMPTOMATIC	21.0	6	600				3.3	5	2	15	3.3	6	7.5	14.0	3.0	7.0	3.0	7.5	6
		17.5	5	450	1.7	10				2	10			5.0	10.5			2.0	10.5	5
III		14.0	4	300	1.7	5				2	5			2.5	7.0	3.0	3.0	2.0	7.0	4
		10.5	3					3.3	0			2.0	3	0	3.5	2.5	2.0	2.0	3.5	3
		7.0	2	150	1.7	0		2.0	0	2	0					2.0	0.0	1.5	0.0	2
IV		3.5	1															1.0	0.0	1

with tests using more standard increments.[4] An exercise test should be individualized so that test duration is approximately 8 to 12 minutes.[1-5]

Recommended Progressive Staged Protocols

Figure 3-2 illustrates three protocols that can be used to cover a wide range of patients. The Bruce is best for relatively fit individuals, whereas the U.S. Air Force School of Aerospace Medicine (USAFSAM) protocols (modifications of the original Balke-Ware) can be used for patients who are less fit. In all of the protocols, stages can be skipped or shortened if the patient adjusts to them quickly to keep the duration to 10 to 12 minutes. The one-half stage can be added to the Bruce for those who find it difficult to use a more physiologic protocol.

Ramp Testing

The ramp protocol, in which work increases constantly and continuously, enables "optimizing" exercise testing because work increments are small and the test is individualized by targeting test duration.[2,6] Figure 3-3 contrasts how the cardiopulmonary system follows the workload (heart rate and $\dot{V}O_2$) in a staged protocol compared with a ramp. Oxygen uptake is overestimated from tests that contain large work increments. In addition, the variability in estimating oxygen uptake from work rate is markedly greater on these tests than for a ramp test. Because this approach appears advantageous, we currently perform all our clinical and research testing using the ramp. If available equipment does not permit ramping, we recommend a modified Balke-Ware protocol such as the USAFSAM. A ramp permits more accurate estimation of aerobic exercise capacity, but otherwise one of the three protocols illustrated in Fig. 3-2 is suitable for most purposes and patients.

Fig. 3-1. The most common protocols, their stages, and the predicted oxygen cost of each stage are illustrated. The associated functional classifications and approximate clinical status are given for comparison. Corresponding METS for ergometer workload are given for a 70-kg person. USAFSAM, U.S. Air Force School of Aerospace Medicine; ACIP, asymptomatic cardiac ischemia pilot; CHF, congestive heart failure (modified Naughton); kpm/min, kilopond meters/minute; % GR, percent grade.

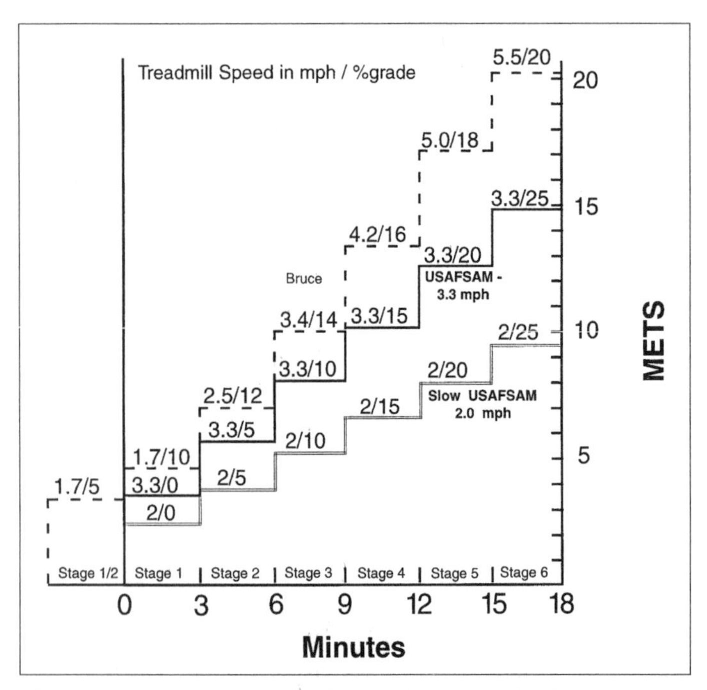

Fig. 3-2. Estimation of METS from three treadmill protocol times or stages. The three protocols can be used to cover a wide range of patients. The Bruce is best for relatively fit individuals, whereas the USAFSAM protocols (modifications of the original Balke-Ware) can be used for patients who are less fit. In all of the protocols, stages can be skipped or shortened if the patient adjusts to them quickly to keep the duration to 10 to 12 minutes. The 1/2 stage can be added to the Bruce protocol. USAFSAM, U.S. Air Force School of Aerospace Medicine.

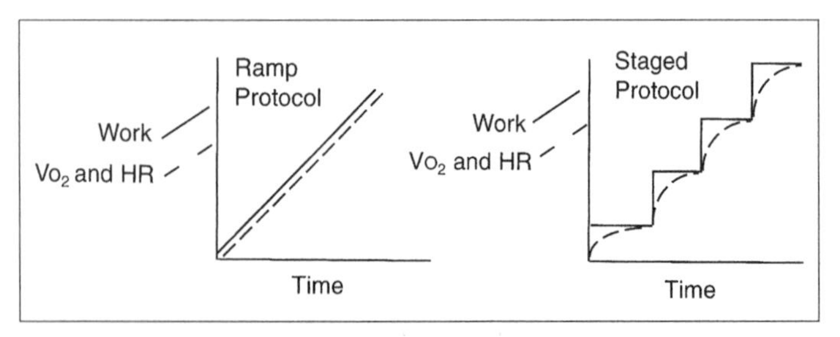

Fig. 3-3. In the ramp protocol, work increases constantly and continuously enabling the exercise test to be optimized since work increments are small and the test is individualized by targeting test duration. This figure contrasts how the cardiopulmonary system follows the workload (heart rate and Vo_2) in a staged protocol compared to a ramp. Oxygen uptake is overestimated from tests which contain large work increments. Special treadmill control software is needed to implement the ramp protocol. HR, heart rate.

REFERENCES

1. Webster MWI, Sharpe DN. Exercise testing in angina pectoris: The importance of protocol design in clinical trials. *Am Heart J* 117:505–508, 1989.
2. Myers J, Buchanan N, Walsh D, Kraemer M, McAuley P, Hamilton-Wessler M, Froelicher VF. Comparison of the ramp versus standard exercise protocols. *J Am Coll Cardiol* 17:1334–1342, 1991.
3. Buchfuhrer MJ, Hansen JE, Robinson TE, Sue DY, Wasserman K, Whipp BJ. Optimizing the exercise protocol for cardiopulmonary assessment. *J Appl Physiol* 55:1558–1564, 1983,
4. Lipkin DP, Canepa-Anson R, Stephens MR, Poole-Wilson PA. Factors determining symptoms in heart failure. Comparison of fast and slow exercise tests. *Br Heart J* 55:439–445, 1986.
5. Myers J, Froelicher VF. Optimizing the exercise test for pharmacological investigations. *Circulation* 1839–1846, 1990.
6. Myers J, Buchanan N, Smith D, Neutel J, Bowes E, Walsh D, Froelicher VF. Individual ramp treadmill: Observations on a new protocol. *Chest* 101:2305–2415, 1992.

Overview of Clinical Exercise Testing

WHO SHOULD HAVE AN EXERCISE TEST?

For Diagnosis

If the diagnosis of coronary artery disease is uncertain, then the exercise test is useful for diagnosing coronary disease. The test should be performed for diagnosis if the patient exhibits any of the following:

Symptoms or signs of coronary artery disease.
Exercise-induced symptoms.
Chest pain.
Old or new ECG abnormalities.

For Prognosis

An exercise test should be performed for prognostication after a recent myocardial infarction (MI) or when angina is stable or has been successfully treated. Because diagnosis has already been determined, the test is used to identify those patients who would benefit from further interventions. The Duke and Veterans Affairs Medical Center (VAMC) Scores can predict cardiac mortality.[1,2]

For Exercise Capacity

When an exercise prescription is required or the degree of disability is uncertain, the test should be done to evaluate exercise capacity. Chronically ill patients diagnosed with diabetes, congestive heart failure (CHF), pulmonary disease, and chronic renal failure are all appropriate candidates for evaluating exercise tolerance. Surgical patients recovering from congenital heart defect repair, valvular replacement, and cardiac transplant can be referred for exercise capacity evaluation.

For Treatment Assessment

The test should be performed to assess treatment if the patient requires testing prior to therapy for baseline measurements or testing after any of the following treatments to demonstrate efficacy:

Medications for angina, arrhythmias, high blood pressure.
Interventions such as percutaneous transluminal coro-

nary angioplasty, coronary artery bypass surgery, and cardiac transplantation.

CONTRAINDICATIONS TO EXERCISE TESTING

It is critical to determine any contraindications to testing before a patient begins testing. A patient may be unable to perform an exercise test because of medical exclusion, inability to walk effectively, or inappropriate or incomplete preparation. If any of these situations occur, testing should be rescheduled (if appropriate) or a nonstress test should be considered.

Medical History

Medical exclusions can be determined through history taking, review of medical records, and physical examination. Factors that increase the risk of testing and can be contraindications are:

Recent complicated MI
Unstable angina
Variant angina
Previous problems with testing, including stability problems or serious cardiac events
Episode of sudden death/ventricular fibrillation requiring treatment
Exercise-induced syncope or arrhythmia
Exacerbation of CHF or evidence for severe left ventricle dysfunction
Obstructive aortic outflow disorder (asymmetric septal hypertrophy, aortic stenosis)
Uncontrolled hypertension
Pericardial tumors or cysts
Cardiac vegetations or endocarditis
Acute pericarditis
Complicating illness or secondary weakness
Instability, vertigo, profound weakness

Questioning and physical examination findings will identify high-risk patients. Specific questions include:

1. Is the patient's disease stable? Are the symptoms stable or unstable (new or increasing symptoms)?
2. Does the patient have true angina pectoris? Question patient regarding any chest pain characteristics and make a determination (i.e., noncardiac, typical, atypical, variant).

3. Outflow obstruction? Listen for systolic murmur and check carotid pulses.
4. Does the patient have CHF? Check the patient's history and tests documenting CHF and examine patient for signs of failure.
5. Has the patient had an MI? Recent or old (test usually should be submaximal if within 3 months, appropriateness determined by MI severity).
6. Is the ECG abnormal? Compare to old ECG if available.
7. What is the patient's CNS status? Stroke or syncopy history?
8. Arrhythmia status? Is there a history of arrhythmia, syncope, sudden death, or cardioversion?

Ambulation

A variety of reasons may explain why the patient is unable to walk effectively on the treadmill. Any assessment of generalized weakness, instability, or vertigo should eliminate use of this test with the patient. If serious deficits from a stroke or other CNS or orthopedic problems limit the patient's ambulation, referral should be made for a nonstress evaluation. A patient with severe claudication usually cannot be tested for diagnosis or prognosis as the response to exercise is limited.

Methodologic Preparation

A patient must be adequately prepared to exercise. The patient must have fasted for 3 hours, been given consent to exercise, and be wearing appropriate clothes for testing. The procedure of the exercise test must be adequately explained along with the chest pain and Borg scale. Equipment must be functioning, and the ECG recording must be free of noise. Emergency equipment must be readily available and a defibrillator should be tested and remain on.

DURING TESTING

Once the patient begins exercise, continual assessment and monitoring begin of the patient's symptoms, ECG response, and hemodynamic variables. The Borg scale is used to assess the level of work while the chest pain scale tracks angina. Blood pressure is recorded every 2 minutes or more frequently if indicated. Continuous ECG monitoring is essential and recording should be done at least every 2 minutes at maximal effort, during immediate recovery, and every minute in recovery (particularly the third minute). Recordings should also be made when serious arrhythmias, a drop in systolic blood pressure, or chest pain occurs.

REASONS FOR TERMINATION

Test termination is dictated by a patient's request, new medical changes, or equipment failure. Listed are the absolute and relative reasons to terminate a test.[3]

Absolute Reasons to Terminate

Acute MI
Severe angina
Exertional hypotension
Serious arrhythmias
Poor perfusion
CNS signs
Technical problems
Patient's request

Relative Reasons to Terminate

More than 3-mm ST shift
Increasing chest pain
Pronounced fatigue and shortness of breath
Wheezing
Leg pain
High blood pressure
Less serious arrhythmia
Bundle branch block that looks like ventricular tachycardia

REFERENCES

1. Morrow K, Morris CK, Froelicher VF, Hideg A, Hunter D, Johnson E, Kawaguchi T, Lehmann K, Ribisl P, Thomas R, Ueshima K, Wallis J. Prediction of cardiovascular death in patients undergoing non-invasive evaluation for coronary artery disease. *Ann Intern Med* 118:689–695, 1993.
2. Mark DB, Hlatky MA, Harrell FE, Lee KL, Califf RM, Pryor DB. Exercise treadmill score for predicting prognosis in coronary artery disease. *Ann Intern Med* 106:793–800, 1987.
3. Fletcher GF, Balady G, Froelicher VF, Hartley LH, Haskell W, Pollack ML. Exercise standards. A statement for healthcare professionals from the American Heart Association. *Circulation* 91:580–615, 1995.

Overview of Exercise Test Interpretation

The objective (exercise capacity, heart rate, blood pressure, ECG changes, and arrhythmias) and subjective (patient appearance, the results of physical examination and symptoms, particularly angina) responses to exercise testing require separate interpretation because each response has a different effect on diagnosis, and clinical decisions and must be considered along with clinical information. A test should not be called abnormal (i.e., a positive test) or normal (i.e., a negative test); rather, the interpretation should specify which responses were normal or abnormal. After interpretation of the exercise test, the application of the results is determined by the initial rationale for testing and prior clinical history.

KEY POINTS FOR INTERPRETATION

1. The variables associated with both perfusion and function abnormalities of the left ventricle (i.e., METS, maximal heart rate, and systolic blood pressure) have the greatest prognostic value.
2. The severity of ischemia or the amount of myocardium in jeopardy is known clinically to be inversely related to the heart rate, blood pressure, and exercise level achieved when ischemia occurs.
3. Neither resting nor exercise ejection fraction (nor its change during exercise) correlate well with measured or estimated maximal ventilatory oxygen uptake, even in patients without signs or symtoms of ischemia.[1] Exercise-induced markers of ischemia do not correlate well with one another.[2]

Variables Considered during Exercise Test Interpretation

Hemodynamics
Exercise capacity
Assessment of effort; if no ST shift or angina occurred, was the effort sufficient to raise myocardial oxygen demand adequately
Symptoms (chest pain should be classified as angina or noncardiac pain or sensation)
Probable presence of clinically significant disease and

probable presence of severe disease (pretest probability combined with an estimate of posttest probability)
ECG (ST shifts and arrhythmias)
Confounders (Wolff-Parkinson-White [WPW], left ventricular hypertrophy [LVH], bundle branch block [BBB], intraventricular conduction defect [IVCD])

Conditions Affecting Interpretation
Were there any existing conditions that affected exercise performance or interpretation of the test?

1. Orthopedic disability.
2. Pulmonary disease? Review pulmonary function test.
3. Obesity? What was the height/weight ratio?
4. CNS disease? What neurologic deficits were present?
5. Deconditioned? Review activity questionnaire.
6. Resting ECG abnormality? When left bundle branch block (LBBB) or WPW are present, ST segment shifts are not associated with ischemia.
7. Resting ST depression or LVH will slightly lessen specificity, but sensitivity remains good. Thus, the exercise ECG still remains the best first diagnostic test.
8. Drugs? Beta blockers can suppress heart rate response; digoxin can effect ST segment shifts.
9. History of CHF? It is associated with limited heart rate rise and decreased exercise capacity.
10. Peripheral vascular disease? Did baseline examination reveal decreased pulses? What distance can the patient normally walk before symptoms occur? Claudication is associated with severe coronary artery disease.

EXERCISE CAPACITY OR FUNCTIONAL CAPACITY

The functional status of patients with heart disease is frequently classified by symptoms during daily activities (New York Heart Association, Canadian, or Weber classifications are common examples). However, there is no substitute for estimated or directly measured maximal ventilatory oxygen uptake. Maximal ventilatory oxygen uptake (Vo_2 max) is the greatest amount of oxygen that a person can extract from inspired air while performing dynamic exercise involving a large part of the total body muscle mass. Because maximal ventilatory oxygen uptake is equal to the product of cardiac output and arterial venous oxygen (a-Vo_2) difference, it is a measure of the functional limits of the cardiovascular system. Maximal a-VO_2 difference is physiologically limited to roughly 15 to 17 volume percent. Thus, maximal a-VO_2 difference behaves more or less as a constant, making maximal oxygen uptake an indirect estimate of maximal cardiac output. In clinical practice, exercise capacity can either be estimated from treadmill speed and grade (see equation in appendix) or measured by analyzing expired gases. Measured expired gases are more accurate since they avoid the problems of hanging on, serial testing, and running vs walking.

METS

For convenience, ventilatory oxygen consumption is expressed in multiples of basal resting requirements (METS). One MET is equal to a unit of basal oxygen consumption measuring approximately 3.5 ml O_2/kg/min. This value is the average oxygen requirement from inspired air to maintain life in the resting state. The maximal MET capacity is dependent on many factors, including natural physical endowment, activity status, age, and gender, but it is the best index of exercise capacity and maximal cardiovascular function. As a rough reference, the maximal oxygen uptake of the normal sedentary adult is approximately 30 ml O_2/kg/min (8.5 METS) and the minimal level for physical fitness is 40 ml O_2/kg/min (11 METS). Aerobic training can increase maximal oxygen uptake by up to 25% and bed rest can do the converse. This increase is dependent on the initial level of fitness and age as well as the intensity, frequency, and length of training sessions. Individuals performing aerobic training such as distance running can have maximal oxygen uptake as high as 60 to 90 ml O_2/kg/min.

A careful review of the literature[3] regarding VO_2 max and its variation with age and activity resulted in a regression equation from 17 previous studies encompassing 700 observations in healthy males of all ages:

$$\text{predicted METS} = 16.2 - 0.11 \text{ (age)}$$

Exercise Capacity and Cardiac Function

Exercise capacity determined by exercise testing has been proposed as a means to estimate ventricular function. A direct relationship would appear to be supported in that both resting ejection fraction (EF) and exercise capacity have prognostic value in patients with coronary heart disease. However, a marked discrepancy between resting ventricular function and exercise performance is frequently seen clinically. In addition, exercise capacity is poorly related to ventricular function in patients with cardiomyopathies. Because exercise-induced ischemia could limit exercise in spite of normal resting ventricular function, patients with angina must be excluded, and silent ischemia must be considered when evaluating an interaction. Resting ventricular function and exercise capacity are both important prognostic features of heart disease, but their association is not highly correlated in patients with stable disease. Because abnormal ventricular function does not imply abnormal exercise capacity in clinical practice, an exercise test must be performed to determine exercise capacity.

METS: Estimated versus Actual

Ventilatory oxygen consumption (MET level) can be estimated from workload or actually measured by gas exchange analysis during treadmill exercise. When MET levels are reported as actual values, a patient has performed a treadmill test while simultaneously measuring expired gases. If MET levels are reported as estimated, the MET level is derived by the amount of work a patient achieves during treadmill testing. The workload is computed by the maximal speed and grade achieved. External work directly correlates to oxygen consumed to achieve the applied work level. This value is estimated by determining the maximum speed and grade achieved and computing total MET level (i.e., max Vo_2). The estimated level is not as accurate as the measured value because of differences in efficiency between patients and hanging on. There are physiologic differences among patients between the match of internal and external work and oxygen kinetics that are only captured by measured Vo_2.

HEART RATE

Maximal Heart Rate

The heart rate response to maximal dynamic exercise is dependent on numerous factors but particularly age and health. Although a regression line of 200 − 0.6 (age) is fairly reproducible, the scatter around this line is considerable (i.e., 1 SD = ± 12 bpm). This makes age-predicted maximal heart rate relatively useless for clinical purposes. Such predictions are maximal for some individuals and submaximal for others.[4]

Methods of Recording

The best way to measure heart rate is to use a standard ECG recorder and use the R-R intervals to calculate instantaneous heart rate. Methods using the arterial pulse or capillary blush technique are much more affected by artifact than electrocardiographic techniques. Some investigators have used averaging over the last minute of exercise or during immediate recovery; both of these methods are inaccurate. Heart rate drops quickly in recovery and can climb steeply even in the last seconds of exercise. Premature beats can affect averaging and must be eliminated to obtain the actual heart rate. Cardiotachometers are available but may fail to trigger or may trigger inappropriately on T-waves, artifact, or aberrant beats, thus yielding inaccurate results.

MEASURES OF MAXIMAL EFFORT

A practical factor determining maximal exercise heart rate is motivation to exert oneself maximally. Older patients may be restrained by poor muscle tone, pulmonary disease, claudication, orthopedic problems, and other noncardiac causes of limitation. The usual decline in maximal heart rate with age is not as steep in persons who are free of myocardial disease and stay active, but it still occurs.

Various objective measurements have been used to confirm that a maximal effort was performed. As maximal aerobic capacity is reached, the rate of oxygen consumption may plateau. A respiratory quotient greater than 1.15, that is, a decrease or failure to increase oxygen uptake by 150 cc/min with increased workloads, is one criterion for the "plateau." However, a plateau is infrequently seen in continuous treadmill protocols in our experience and may actually be due to holding onto the handrails, incomplete expired air collection, the criteria used for plateau, differences in the sampling interval, or the equipment used.[5]

The Borg scale has been developed to grade subjectively levels of exertion. This method is best applied to match levels of perceived exertion during comparison studies. The linear scale ranges from 6 (very, very light) to 20 (very, very hard), the nonlinear scale ranges from 0 to 10, and both correlate with the percentage of maximal heart rate during exercise. Respiratory quotient, the ratio of carbon dioxide production to oxygen uptake, increases in proportion to exercise effort. Values of 1.15 are reached by most individuals at the point of maximal dynamic exercise. However, this varies greatly and requires gas exchange analysis during exercise. Lactic acid levels have also been used (i.e., >7 or 8 mMol), but they also require mixed venous samples and vary greatly among individuals.

BLOOD PRESSURE RESPONSE

Systolic blood pressure (SBP) should rise with increasing treadmill workload. Diastolic blood pressure usually remains about the same, but the fifth Korotkoff sound can sometimes be heard all the way to zero in healthy young subjects. Systolic blood pressure rises to about twice its resting value during dynamic exercise, whereas normally diastolic blood pressure drops or stays the same. Although a rising diastolic blood pressure can be associated with coronary heart disease, it is more likely a marker for labile hypertension, which leads to coronary disease. The highest systolic blood pressure should be achieved at maximal workload. When exercise is stopped, approximately 10% of the people tested will abruptly drop their SBP owing to peripheral pooling. To avoid fainting, patients should not be left standing on the treadmill. Systolic blood pressure usually normalizes on resuming the supine position within 3 to 5 minutes during recovery but may remain below normal for several hours after the test. In spite of studies showing discrepancies between noninvasively and invasively measured blood pressure, the product of heart rate and SBP, determined by cuff and auscultation, correlates with measured myocardial oxygen consumption during exercise. It should be emphasized that the automated methods of measuring SBP have not proven to be accurate. Although the available devices may correlate with manual methods, they have not yet been adequately validated, particularly for the detection of exertional hypotension.

Double Product

The double product, heart rate times SBP, is an index of myocardial oxygen consumption. An individual patient's angina pectoris will be precipitated at the same double product. This product is also an estimate of the maximal workload that the left ventricle can perform.

Exertional Hypotension

Exercise-induced hypotension (EIH) has been demonstrated in most studies to predict either a poor prognosis or a high probability of severe angiographic coronary artery disease. Although the prognosis for patients with EIH has not been specifically examined after myocardial infarction, an abnormal systolic blood pressure response has been found to indicate an increased risk for cardiac events in this population. In addition, EIH has been associated with cardiac complications during exercise testing and appears to be corrected by coronary artery bypass surgery.[6-7]

The normal blood pressure response to dynamic upright exercise consists of a progressive increase in SBP, no change or a decrease in diastolic blood pressure, and a widening of the pulse pressure. Even when tested to exhaustion, healthy individuals do not exhibit a reduction in SBP of any kind. Normally, after exercise, there is a drop in both systolic and diastolic pressure. Exercise-induced decreases in SBP (EIH) can occur in patients with coronary artery disease, valvular heart disease, cardiomyopathies, and arrhythmias. Occasionally, patients without clinically significant heart disease will exhibit EIH during exercise due to antihypertensive therapy including beta blockers, prolonged strenuous exercise, or vasovagal responses. It can also occur in healthy females. Pathophysiologically, EIH could be due to chronic ventricular dysfunction, exercise-induced ischemia causing left ventricular dysfunction, or papillary muscle dysfunction and mitral regurgitation. Exercise-induced hypotension is usually related to myocardial ischemia or myocardial infarction, is best defined as a drop in SBP during exercise below the standing preexercise value, and indicates a significantly increased risk of cardiac events. This increased risk is not found in those who did not have either a prior myocardial infarction or signs or symptoms of ischemia during the exercise test. It is usually associated with three-vessel or left main coronary artery disease. Although EIH appears to be reversed by revascularization procedures, confirmation of a beneficial effect on survival requires a randomized trial.

PRETEST PROBABILITY OF CORONARY DISEASE

There are tables and equations that can be used to estimate the probability of an individual having coronary artery disease. These are based on age, gender, risk factors (serum cholesterol, blood pressure, smoking) and risk markers (ECG, family history). However, the most meaningful and practical alterations in probability in those in whom coronary disease is most prevalent are caused by symptomatology. Any history of a cardiac event (i.e., myocardial infarction) or symptoms of ischemia (angina) drastically raise the pretest probability. Typical angina pectoris or a myocardial infarction is associated with a 90% probability of significant coronary disease and atypical angina with a 50% probability in a middle-aged male. These estimates should be used for deciding if the test is indicated and what the posttest probability of disease is after the test results are known.

ST ANALYSIS

Interpretation of the exercise ECG is critical to proper use of the exercise test. Certain key points will be illustrated below in algorithms and flow diagrams. Figure 5-1 illustrates the normal ECG response to treadmill exercise. Note that there can be considerable normal ST junctional (junction of the QRS and ST wave forms) depression.

Measurement Point

The ST level should be measured at the end of the QRS complex, which is the beginning of the ST segment. It is best to determine this point by considering QRS activity in three dimensions as the QRS complex can appear flat in some leads while it is still on-going in others. Other terms for this point are the **J-junction** and **ST0** (i.e., the junction between the QRS complex and ST segment, 0 msec after QRS).

Isoelectric Reference Line

The zero reference point at which the isoelectric line is set for wave form amplitudes is the **PQ point.** This is the point between the end of atrial depolarization (P wave) and the onset of the Q wave. It can be distorted by short PR intervals and atrial repolarization. Computer programs frequently miss this level, resulting in erroneous ST amplitude calculations.

ST Shift Amplitudes

The ST response that should be measured depends on whether the response is elevation or depression based on the standing ST level. The standing ST levels are illustrated in Figs. 5-2, 5-3, and 5-4. The standing ST level can

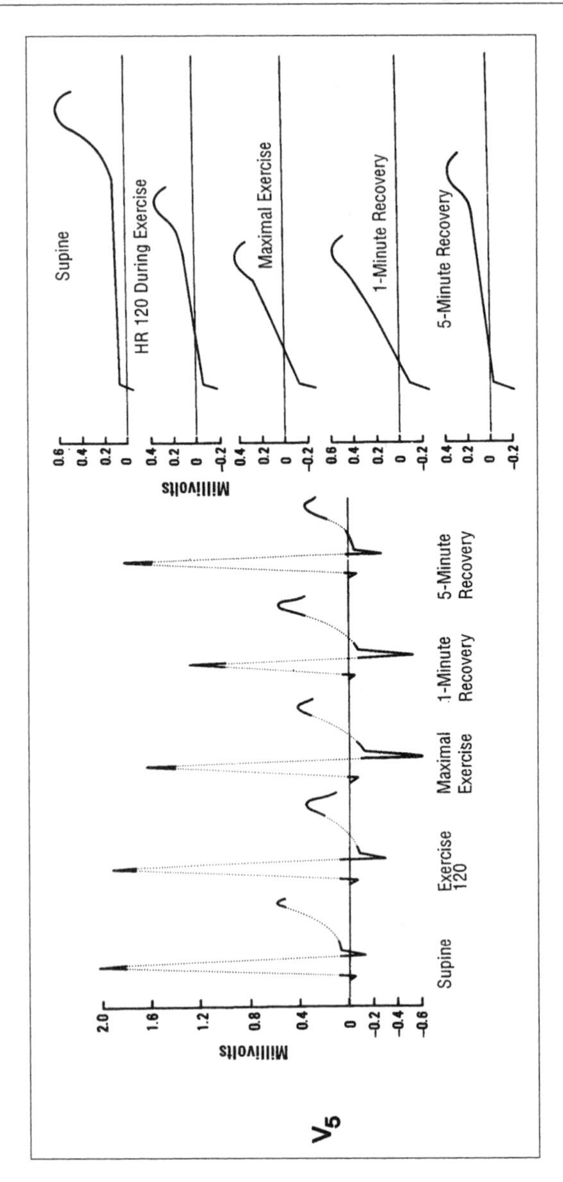
V5
Millivolts
2.0
1.6
1.2
0.8
0.4
0
−0.2
−0.4
−0.6
Supine
Exercise 120
Maximal Exercise
1-Minute Recovery
5-Minute Recovery
Millivolts
Supine
HR 120 During Exercise
Maximal Exercise
1-Minute Recovery
5-Minute Recovery

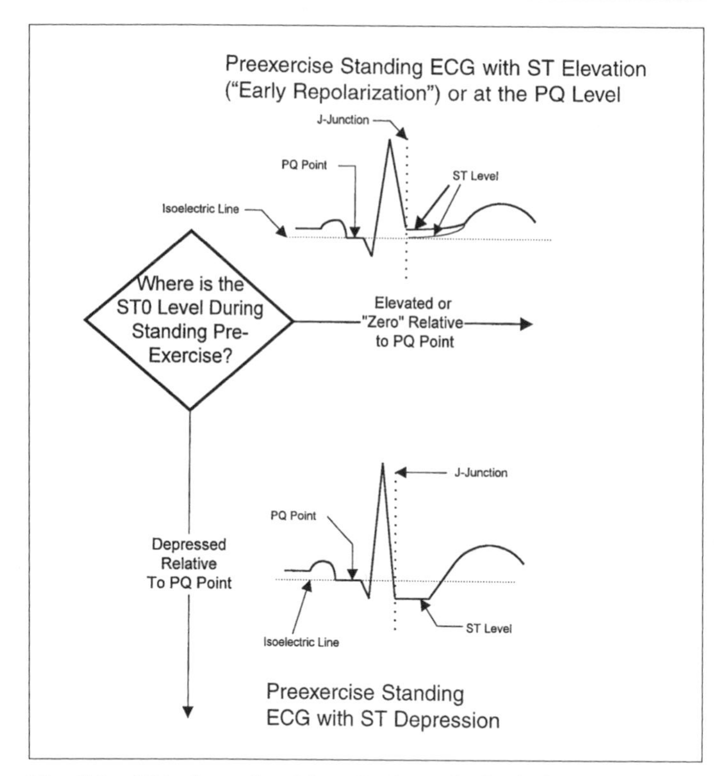

Fig. 5-2. This flow algorithm displays the logic for measuring the ST response to exercise. The ST measurement depends on whether the response is elevation or depression based on the standing ST level. The standing ST level at the top of the illustration is elevated (on or above the isoelectric line). See Fig. 5-3 for an illustration of how the ST segment changes with exercise are measured with this circumstance. The standing ST level at the top of the illustration is depressed. See Fig. 5-4 for an illustration of how the ST segment changes with exercise are measured with this circumstance.

be elevated, depressed, or zero. The exercise responses are illustrated in Figs. 5-4 and 5-5. Elevation is measured from the standing ST level, and the criterion is 0.5 mm without slope considered. Depression is measured from the isoelectric PQ point whether the standing ST segment is elevated (early repolarization) or on the isoelectric line. The criteria must consider slope (as determined over the 60 msec after QRS end), with flat being abnormal and downsloping worse. Upsloping is never abnormal but borderline if the ST segment is still depressed by 2 mm or

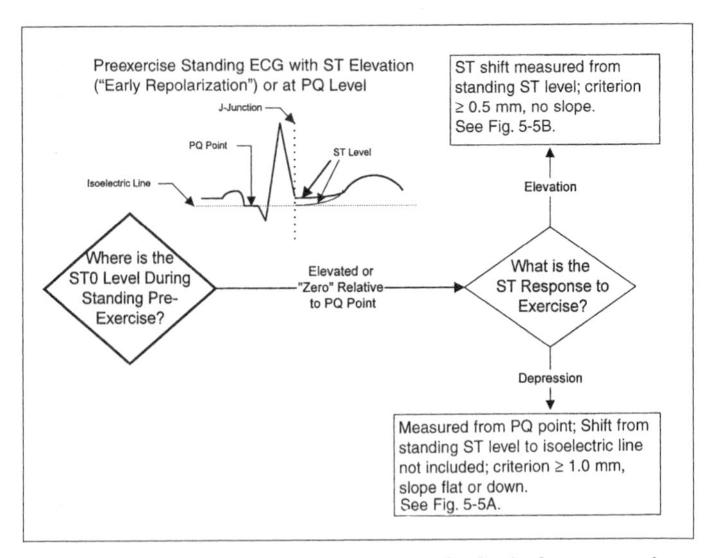

Fig. 5-3. This flow algorithm displays the logic for measuring the ST response for exercise. The ST measurement depends on whether the response is elevation or depression based on the standing ST level. The standing ST level illustrated in Fig. 5-2 is on the isoelectric line or elevated (i.e., early repolarization). Elevation is measured from the standing ST level, and the criterion is 0.5 mm without slope considered. Depression is measured from the level of ST depression.

more at 60 msec after QRS end. These criteria are illustrated in Fig. 5-6.

INTERPRETATION USING EXERCISE TEST VARIABLES

Consideration of exercise test variables (HR, SBP, METS, ECG response), baseline and exercise symptoms, and pretest probability is required for making the diagnosis of coronary artery disease. Applying algorithms that use these variables allows the clinician to estimate the probability of coronary artery disease presence and severity as well as the risk of cardiovascular death. These variables are mathematically incorporated into the prognostic scores and diagnostic algorithms. The VAMC and Duke scores are used for determining prognosis in all patients with stable coronary disease and in patients 6 months after myocardial infarction.[8-9] There is no score available for patients less than 6 months after myocardial infarction.

MET levels can be compared to those of age-matched

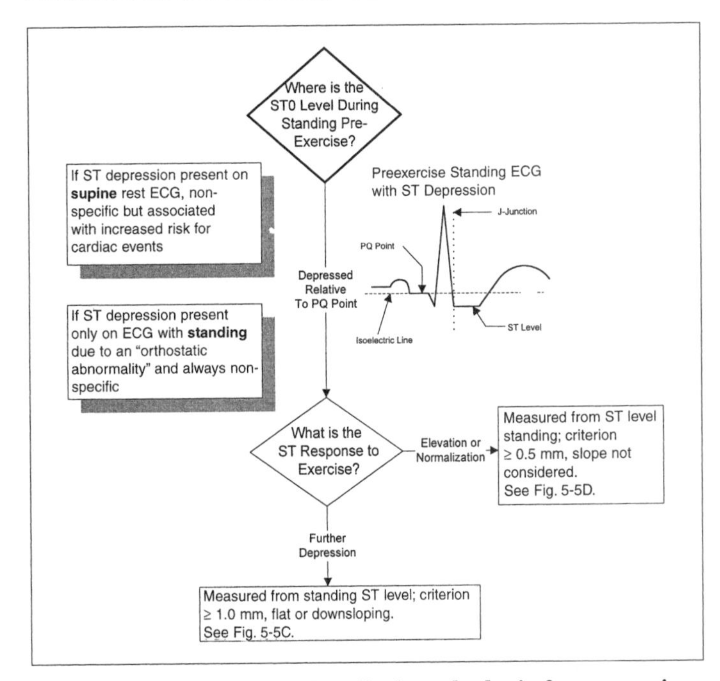

Fig. 5-4. This flow algorithm displays the logic for measuring the ST response to exercise. The ST measurement depends on whether the response is elevation or depression based on the standing ST level. The standing ST level illustrated in Fig. 5-4 is depressed. Elevation is measured from the standing ST level, and the criteria is 0.5 mm without slope considered. Depression is measured from the level of ST depression.

normals according to activity status. Nomograms have been based on regression equations to facilitate the description of exercise capacity relative to age and enable comparison between patients. Reporting exercise capacity as a percentage, with 100% as normal for age, is a useful means of assessing a patient's cardiovascular status.[10] The following general MET levels are also useful:

1 MET = basal level

2–4 METS = 2 to 4 miles per hour walking on level ground

5 METS = activities of daily living; if maximal, associated with poor prognosis; the usual limit set immediately after myocardial infarction

10 METS = a fit, very active individual and associated with a good prognosis

20 METS = aerobic athlete

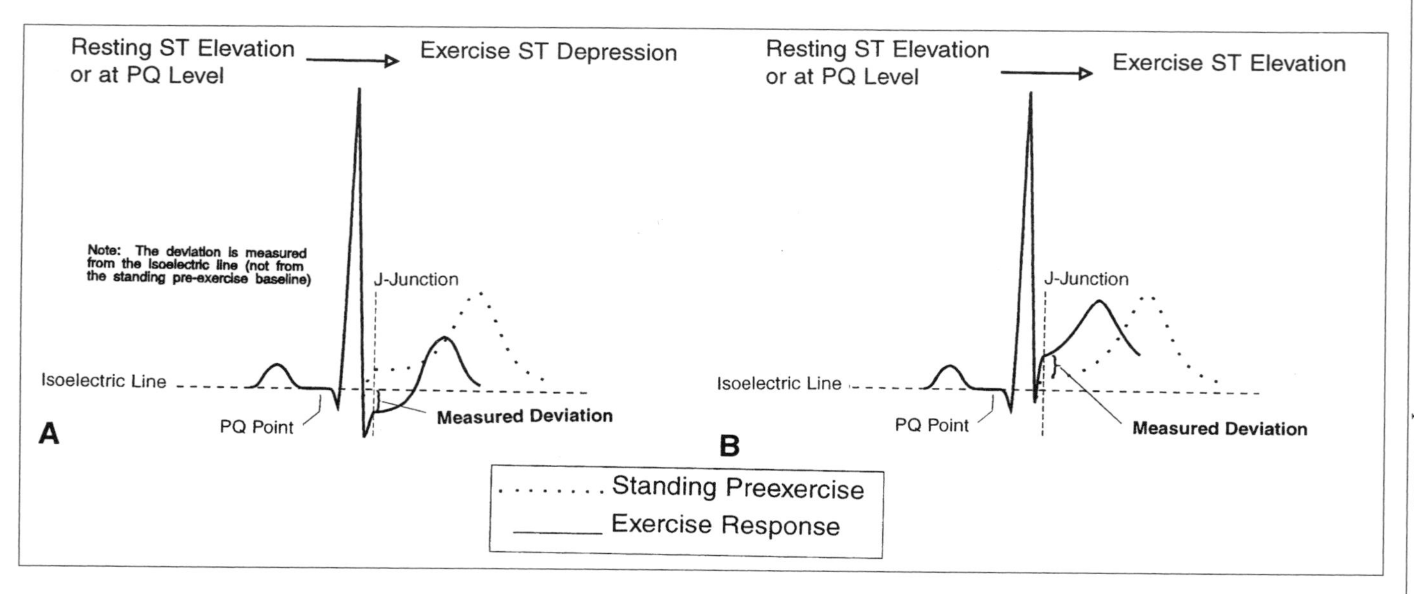
Resting ST Elevation or at PQ Level
Exercise ST Depression
Note: The deviation is measured from the isoelectric line (not from the standing pre-exercise baseline)
J-Junction
Isoelectric Line
PQ Point
Measured Deviation
A
Resting ST Elevation or at PQ Level
Exercise ST Elevation
J-Junction
Isoelectric Line
PQ Point
Measured Deviation
B
Standing Preexercise
Exercise Response

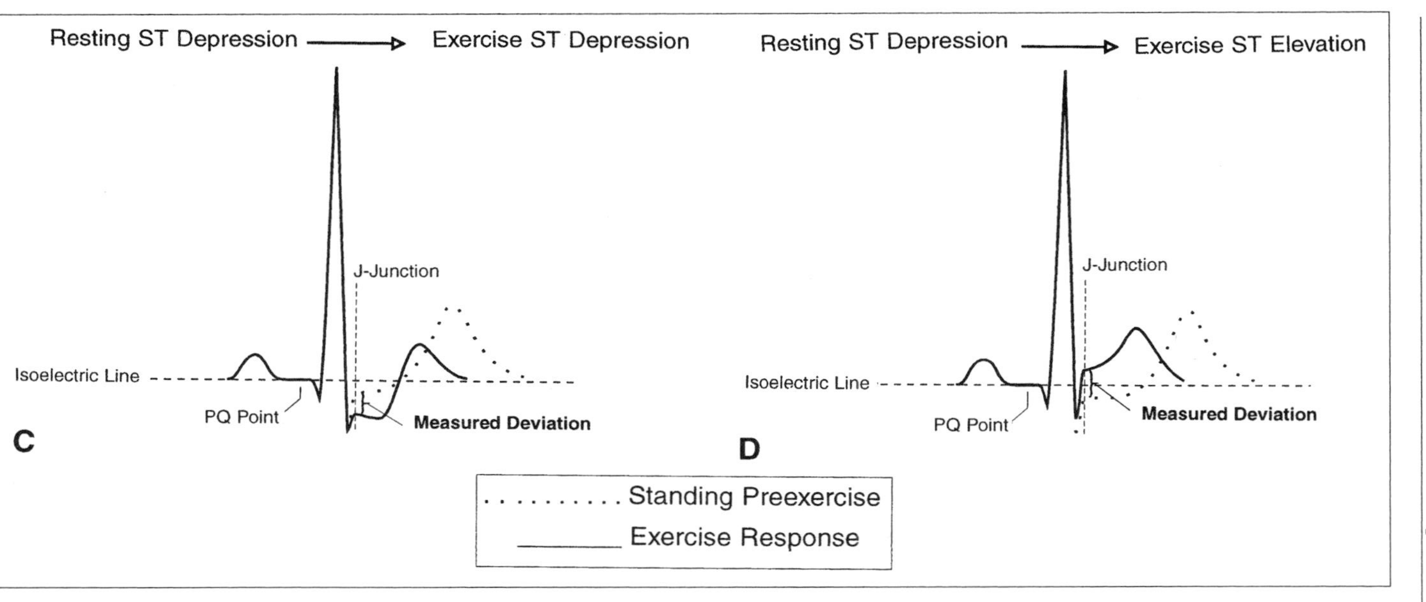
Resting ST Depression → Exercise ST Depression
Resting ST Depression → Exercise ST Elevation
J-Junction
Isoelectric Line
PQ Point
Measured Deviation
C
J-Junction
Isoelectric Line
PQ Point
Measured Deviation
D
Standing Preexercise
Exercise Response

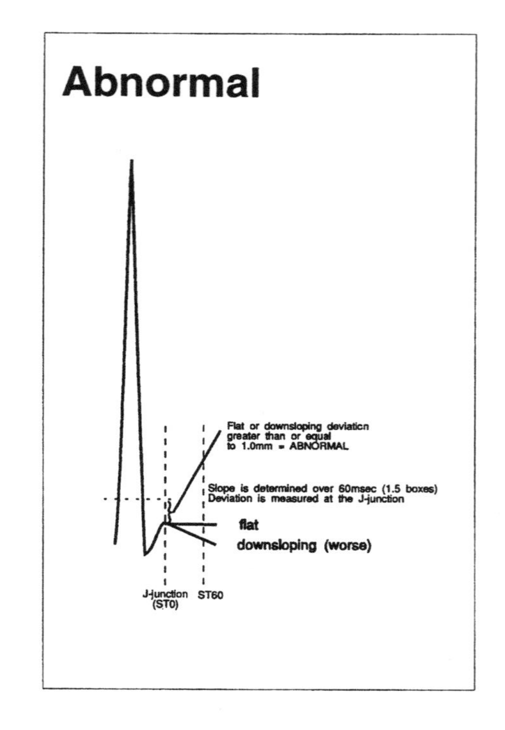
Abnormal
Flat or downsloping deviation greater than or equal to 1.0mm = ABNORMAL
Slope is determined over 60msec (1.5 boxes)
Deviation is measured at the J-junction
flat
downsloping (worse)
J-junction (ST0)
ST60

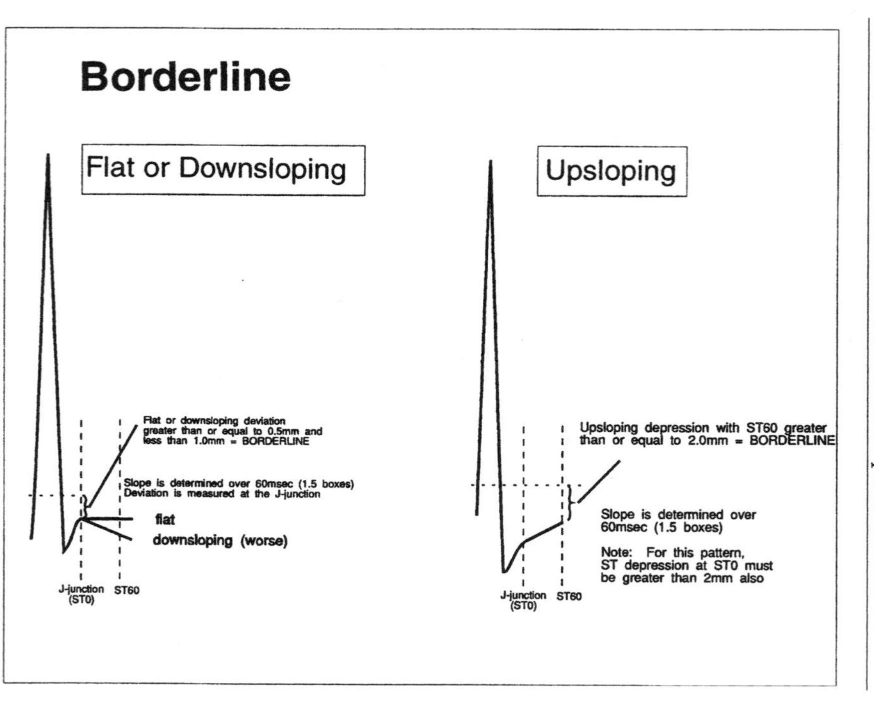
Borderline
Flat or Downsloping
Flat or downsloping deviation greater than or equal to 0.5mm and less than 1.0mm = BORDERLINE
Slope is determined over 60msec (1.5 boxes)
Deviation is measured at the J-junction
flat
downsloping (worse)
J-junction (ST0)
ST60
Upsloping
Upsloping depression with ST60 greater than or equal to 2.0mm = BORDERLINE
Slope is determined over 60msec (1.5 boxes)
Note: For this pattern, ST depression at ST0 must be greater than 2mm also
J-junction (ST0)
ST60

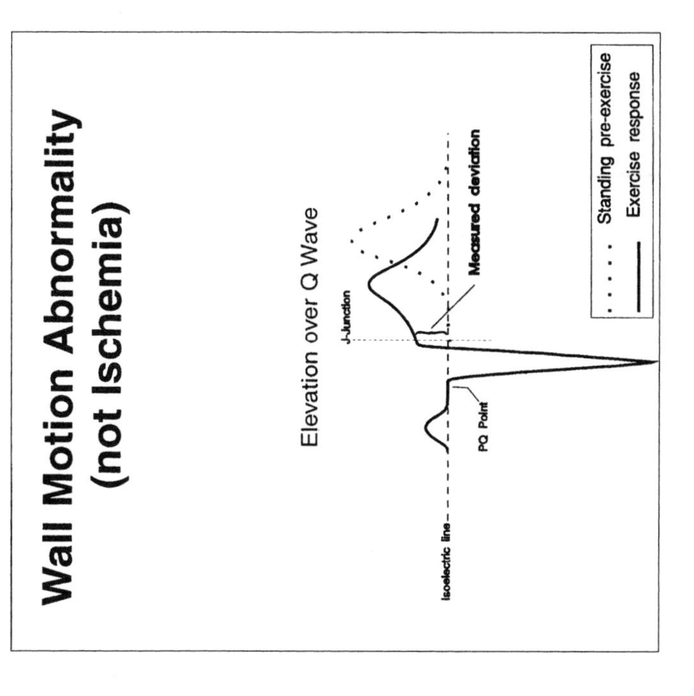
Wall Motion Abnormality
(not Ischemia)
Elevation over Q Wave
J-Junction
Measured deviation
PQ Point
Isoelectric line
Standing pre-exercise
Exercise response

REFERENCES

1. McKirnan MD, Sullivan M, Jensen D, Froelicher VF. Treadmill performance and cardiac function in selected patients with coronary heart disease. *J Am Coll Cardiol* 3:253–261, 1984.
2. Hammond HK, Kelley TL, Froelicher VF. Noninvasive testing in the evaluation of myocardial ischemia: Agreement among tests. *J Am Coll Cardiol* 5:59–69, 1985.
3. Dehn MM, Bruce RA. Longitudinal variations in maximal oxygen intake with age and activity. *J Appl Physiol* 33:805–807, 1972.
4. Hammond K, Froelicher VF. Normal and abnormal heart rate responses to exercise. *Prog Cardiovasc Dis* 27:271–296, 1985.
5. Myers J, Walsh D, Buchanan N, Froelicher VF. Can maximal cardiopulmonary capacity be recognized by a plateau of oxygen uptake? *Chest* 96:1312–1316, 1989.
6. Thomson PD, Kelemen MH. Hypotension accompanying the onset of exertional angina. *Circulation* 52: 28–32, 1975.
7. Dubach P, Froelicher VF, Klein J, Oakes D, Grover-McKay M, Friis R. Exercise-induced hypotension in a male population—criteria, causes, and prognosis. *Circulation* 78:1380–1387, 1988.
8. Morrow K, Morris CK, Froelicher VF, Hideg A, Hunter D, Johnson E, Kawaguchi T, Lehmann K, Ribisl P, Thomas R, Ueshima K, Wallis J. Prediction of cardiovascular death in patients undergoing noninvasive evaluation for coronary artery disease. *Ann Intern Med* 118:689–695, 1993.
9. Mark DB, Hlatky MA, Harrell FE, Lee KL, Califf RM, Pryor DB. Exercise treadmill score for predicting prognosis in coronary artery disease. *Ann Intern Med* 106:793–800, 1987.
10. Morris CK, Myers J, Froelicher VF, Kawaguchi T, Ueshima K, Hideg A. Nomogram for exercise capacity using METs and age. *J Am Coll Cardiol* 22:175–182, 1993.

Key Points from Part I

A major increase and redistribution of cardiac output underlie a series of adjustments that allow the body to increase its resting metabolic rate as much as 10 to 20 times with exercise. The capacity of the body to deliver and use oxygen is expressed as the maximal oxygen uptake. Maximal oxygen uptake is defined as the product of maximal cardiac output and maximal arteriovenous oxygen difference. Thus, the cardiopulmonary limits are defined by (1) a central component (cardiac output), which describes the capacity of the heart to function as a pump; (2) peripheral factors (arteriovenous oxygen difference), which describes the capacity of the lung to oxygenate the blood delivered to it; and (3) the capacity of the working muscle to extract this oxygen from the blood. Hemodynamic response to exercise is greatly affected by the type of exercise being performed; whether disease is present; and the age, gender, and fitness of the individual.

The transport of oxygen from the air to the mitochondria of the working muscle cell requires the coupling of blood flow and ventilation to cellular metabolism. Energy for muscular contraction is provided by three sources: stored phosphates (adenosine triphosphate [ATP], creatinine phosphokinase [CP], oxygen-independent glycolysis, and oxidative metabolism. Oxidative metabolism provides the greatest source of ATP for muscular contraction. Muscular contraction is accomplished by three fiber types that differ in their contraction speed, color, and mitochondrial content. The duration and intensity of activity determine the extent to which these fuel sources and fiber types are needed.

Coronary artery disease reduces myocardial oxygen supply, which, in the presence of an increased myocardial oxygen demand, can lead to myocardial ischemia and reduced cardiac performance. Although myocardial perfusion and function are intuitively linked, it is often difficult to separate the effect of ischemia from that of left ventricular dysfunction on exercise responses. Indices of ventricular function and exercise capacity are poorly related. Cardiac output is considered the most important determinant of exercise capacity in healthy subjects. However, among patients with heart disease, abnormalities in one or several of the links in the chain that define oxygen uptake interact to determine exercise capacity.

Because it can objectively demonstrate exercise capacity, exercise testing is used for disability evaluation rather than relying on functional classifications. Questionnaires or submaximal tests or nonexercise stress tests cannot give the same results as a symptom-limited exercise test. Age-predicted maximal heart rate targets are relatively useless for clinical purposes, and it is surprising how much steeper the age-related decline in maximal heart rate is in referred populations compared with age-matched healthy subjects or volunteers. A consistent finding in population studies has been a relatively poor relationship of maximal heart rate to age. Correlation coefficients of −0.4 are usually found with a standard error of the estimate of 10 to 25 bpm. In general, this has not been "tightened" by considering activity status, weight, cardiac size, maximal respiratory quotient, or perceived exertion.

Exertional hypotension, best defined as a drop in systolic blood pressure to less than standing rest, is very predictive of severe angiographic coronary artery disease and a poor prognosis. A failure of systolic blood pressure to rise is particularly worrisome after a myocardial infarction. Because of the limitations of automated devices, blood pressure should be taken manually with a cuff and stethoscope. This is not difficult after practice.

Nomograms facilitate the description of exercise capacity relative to age and enable comparison between patients. Reporting exercise capacity as a percentage, with 100% as normal for age, has many advantages. Exercise capacity relative to the peers in an age group is a useful means of assessing a patient's cardiovascular status. In addition, patients themselves seem to have a better understanding of this concept. METS is a term that can improve communication between physicians, whereas percent normal exercise capacity can do the same for dialogue between physicians and their patients.

Conducting the Test

Conducting the Test

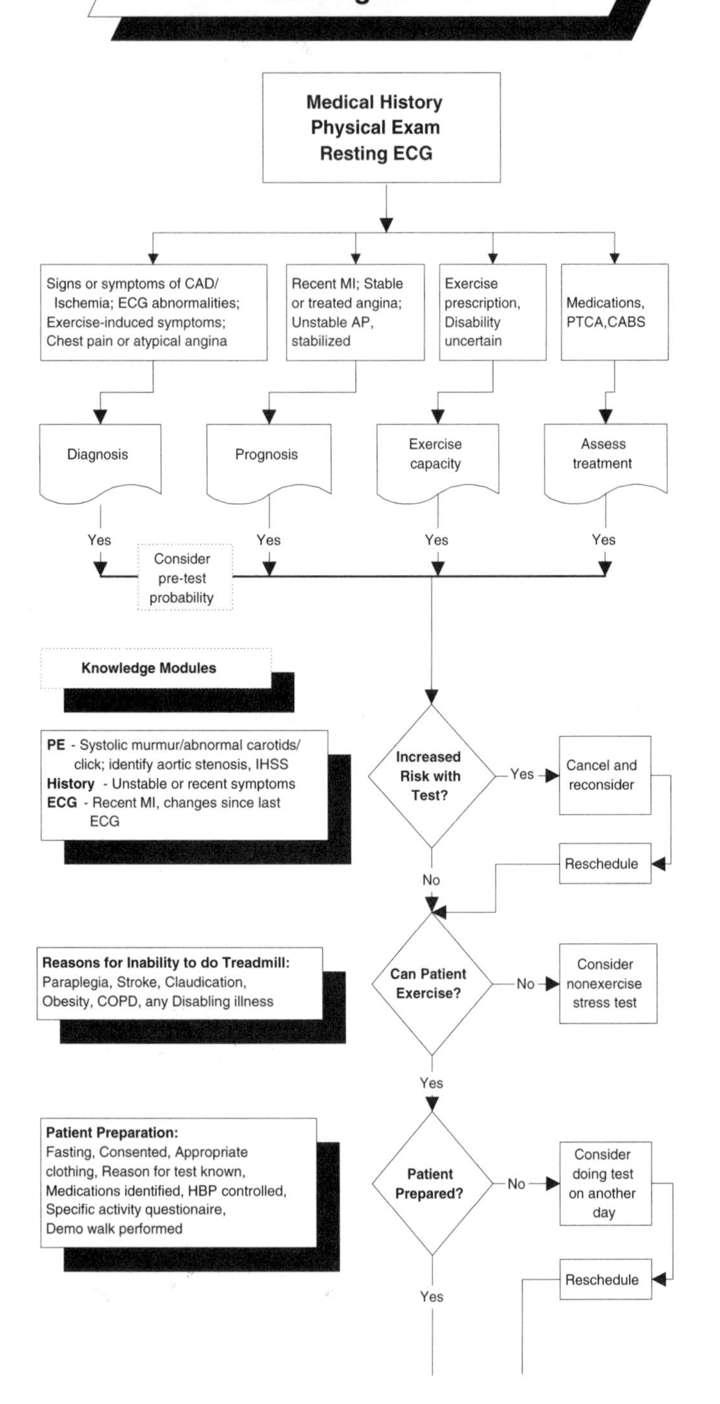

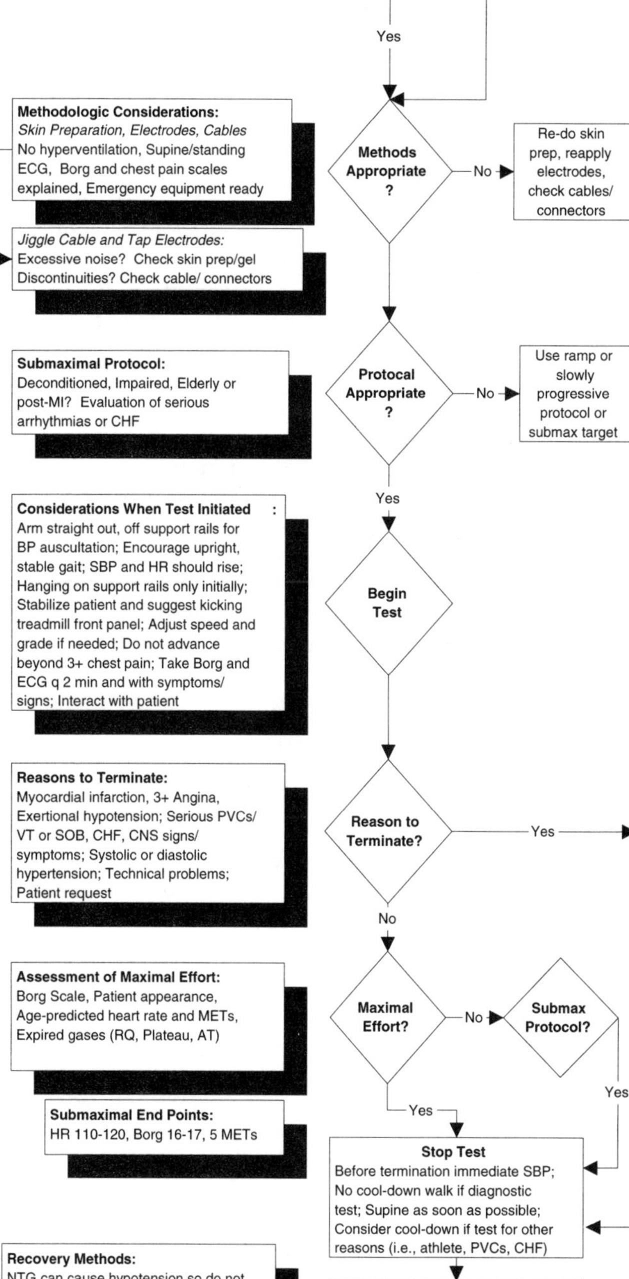
Yes
Methodologic Considerations:
Skin Preparation, Electrodes, Cables
No hyperventilation, Supine/standing ECG, Borg and chest pain scales explained, Emergency equipment ready
Methods Appropriate ?
No
Re-do skin prep, reapply electrodes, check cables/ connectors
Jiggle Cable and Tap Electrodes:
Excessive noise? Check skin prep/gel
Discontinuities? Check cable/ connectors
Submaximal Protocol:
Deconditioned, Impaired, Elderly or post-MI? Evaluation of serious arrhythmias or CHF
Protocal Appropriate ?
No
Use ramp or slowly progressive protocol or submax target
Yes
Considerations When Test Initiated :
Arm straight out, off support rails for BP auscultation; Encourage upright, stable gait; SBP and HR should rise; Hanging on support rails only initially; Stabilize patient and suggest kicking treadmill front panel; Adjust speed and grade if needed; Do not advance beyond 3+ chest pain; Take Borg and ECG q 2 min and with symptoms/ signs; Interact with patient
Begin Test
Reasons to Terminate:
Myocardial infarction, 3+ Angina, Exertional hypotension; Serious PVCs/ VT or SOB, CHF, CNS signs/ symptoms; Systolic or diastolic hypertension; Technical problems; Patient request
Reason to Terminate?
Yes
No
Assessment of Maximal Effort:
Borg Scale, Patient appearance, Age-predicted heart rate and METs, Expired gases (RQ, Plateau, AT)
Maximal Effort?
No
Submax Protocol?
Yes
Submaximal End Points:
HR 110-120, Borg 16-17, 5 METs
Yes
Stop Test
Before termination immediate SBP; No cool-down walk if diagnostic test; Supine as soon as possible; Consider cool-down if test for other reasons (i.e., athlete, PVCs, CHF)
Recovery Methods:
NTG can cause hypotension so do not administer; Monitor ECG for at least 5 min or until changes stabilize; Always record 3 min post-exercise ECG since it is very important; Sit patient up if Severe Ischemia, CHF, or PVCs occur
Recovery
Supine, monitor SBP, symptoms and ECG each minute for 5 min; Emergency procedures as needed; If new ST depression occurs, monitor ECG until the changes stabilize

Initial Evaluation

BASELINE DATA

1. The exercise test should be an extension of the history and physical examination, which must be completed prior to exercising a referred patient.
2. A physician obtains the most information by interviewing, observing, and examining the patient in conjunction with the test.
3. The physician's reaction to signs or symptoms should be moderated by the information the patient gives regarding usual activities. If abnormal findings occur at levels of exercise that the patient usually performs, then it may not be necessary to stop the test for them. Also, the patient's activity history should help determine appropriate workloads for testing.
4. Initial evaluation includes history, physical examination, and ECG review. An attempt should be made to obtain and review prior medical records.

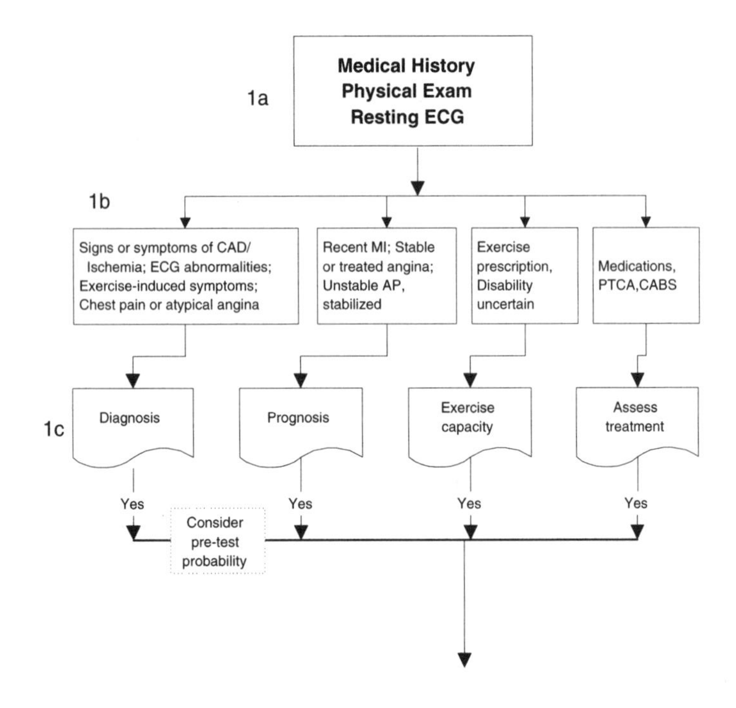

History

The history should include the following:

1. History of current illness: chest pain pattern, dyspnea on exertion (DOE), paroxysmal nocturnal dyspnea (PND), change in weight, palpitations, loss of consciousness, leg or abdominal swelling.
2. Past medical history: usual activities, hospitalizations, illnesses and injuries, cigarette and alcohol use, medications, results of prior tests, myocardial infarction (MI), angina, surgery, substance abuse, and cerebrovascular accidents (CVA).
3. Review of systems: head, eyes; pulmonary; cardiovascular; gastrointestinal; genitourinary; renal; hematologic; orthopedic; and neurologic.
4. Family history: the usual items, plus coronary heart disease in those younger than 65 years, sudden death, and hyperlipidemia.

Physical Examination

1. A minimal cardiovascular examination should include vital signs, assessment of carotids, jugular venous pulse, lungs, heart, abdomen, extremities, and peripheral pulses. The main goal of the examination should be to identify or rule out significant obstructive aortic valvular disease, obstructive or nonobstructive cardiomyopathy, and dilated cardiomyopathy.
2. A neurologic examination should be performed if deficits are suspected from the patient's appearance or from the history. Observing the patient walk is particularly helpful.
3. A systolic murmur accompanied by delayed carotid pulses may necessitate an echocardiogram prior to testing.

Resting ECG

1. The baseline data include the interpretation of the supine ECG and comparison with prior ECG. New symptoms and ECG changes could require postponement of the test. Left bundle branch block and Wolff-Parkinson-White make ST analysis invalid for ischemia.
2. The standing ECG is only used for comparative ST analysis if the standing position causes the ST segments to drop below the PQ isoelectric level.

CATEGORIES FOR EXERCISE TESTING

1. Exercise testing is used to determine the patient's physiologic response to exercise under a medically supervised situation.
2. There are four principal reasons for exercise testing: diagnosis, prognosis, exercise capacity, and treatment assessment.
3. The reason for testing should be clear to the patient and to the physician before performing the test.

Diagnosis

Diagnosis of coronary artery disease is a common request for referral to exercise testing. Specific rules for a positive or abnormal test and cofounders causing false positives must be considered while interpreting results. Pretest probability also influences the usefulness of the test and the likelihood that the test results are true. Although the most common diagnostic issue is whether significant coronary disease or ischemia is present, less common diagnostic uses include testing the hemodynamic significance of valvular disease and assessing whether exercise-induced symptoms are due to arrhythmias.

Prognosis

There are two principal reasons for estimating prognosis. The first is to provide accurate answers to patients' questions regarding the probable outcome of their illness. Most patients find this information useful in planning their affairs regarding work, recreational activities, personal estate, and finances. The second reason to estimate prognosis is to identify patients in whom interventions might improve outcome. The exercise test has been demonstrated to be of value for estimating prognosis, not only in patients with stable symptoms but also in new patients, such as those with uncompleted infarctions due to thrombolytic therapy, those with non-Q-wave myocardial infarctions, and those who have had unstable angina. Scores and metaanalyses have led to a much more scientific estimate of prognosis from exercise test data.

Exercise Capacity Evaluation

Exercise testing is also performed to evaluate a patient's exercise capacity. The information obtained can allow the health care provider to institute or reevaluate an exercise prescription. Disabilities can be clarified with exercise testing and can be monitored through serial testing. Surgical patients recovering from congenital heart defect repair, valvular replacement, and cardiac transplant can be referred for exercise capacity evaluation. Other chronically ill patients evaluated for exercise capacity include those with congestive heart failure, diabetes, chronic renal failure, and pulmonary disease.

Treatment Assessment

The exercise test can be used to evaluate the effects of medical or surgical treatment. The effects of various medications for angina, congestive heart failure, and hypertension, including nitrates, digitalis, and antihypertensive agents, have been evaluated by exercise testing. Exercise testing has also been used to evaluate patients before and after coronary artery bypass surgery (CABS), percutaneous transluminal coronary angioplasty (PTCA), and cardiac transplantation.

PRETEST PROBABILITY/DISEASE SEVERITY

Standard risk factors or markers do not increase the probability of coronary disease to any degree so profoundly as the patient's symptoms of chest pain. For instance, it has been demonstrated that even hypercholesterolemia does not increase the pretest probability enough to make exercise testing cost-effective for screening asymptomatic men. Atypical angina, however, raises the pretest probability for significant angiographic coronary disease to 50% in a middle-aged male, whereas typical angina raises it to 90%. The respective probabilities for severe coronary disease with these symptoms are approximately 25% and 50%, respectively. Although lesser probabilities are associated with younger ages and the female gender, these values apply to most patients being initially evaluated for coronary disease.

Contraindications to Testing

Before initiating an exercise test, contraindications to exercise testing must be addressed. If any contraindications are present, the patient should either be rescheduled for later testing or referred to another evaluation method.

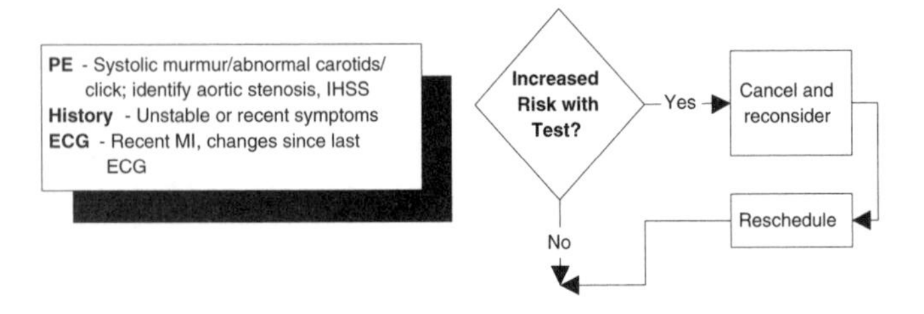

INCREASED RISK

Contraindications increasing a patient's risk can be identified from the history, physical examination, or ECG findings. Specific questions from the history intake would include the following:

1. Is the patient's disease stable? Are the symptoms stable or unstable (new or increasing symptoms)?
2. Does the patient have true angina pectoris? Question the patient regarding any chest pain characteristics and make a determination (i.e., is it noncardiac, typical, atypical variant?).
3. Does the patient have congestive heart failure (CHF)? Check the patient's history and tests documenting CHF.
4. What is the patient's neurologic status? Is there a history of stroke or syncope?
5. Arrhythmia status? Is there a history of palpitations, arrhythmias, syncope, sudden death, or cardioversion?
6. Is there a history of uncontrolled hypertension?

The following questions identify the contraindications to testing:

1. A brief physical examination should always be performed to rule out significant obstructive aortic valvular disease, obstructive or nonobstructive cardiomyopathy, and dilated cardiomyopathy.
2. If a patient is diagnosed with dilated cardiomyopathy, signs of CHF and left ventricular dysfunction should

be noted. If a patient has decompensated from heart failure or from a recent myocardial infarction (MI), the test should not be performed.

3. If the patient has aortic stenosis by history and examination, an echocardiogram, including a doppler assessment of the aortic gradient, should usually be obtained.
4. A baseline supine ECG should be compared with a previous ECG to determine significant changes and baseline abnormalities.
5. Myocardial infarction status, new or old and its severity, determines whether the test should use a maximal or submaximal protocol.

Following is a summary of factors that increase the risk of testing and can be contraindications:

Recent MI
Unstable angina
Variant angina
Previous problems with testing
Episode of sudden death/ventricular tachycardia requiring treatment
Exercise-induced syncope or arrhythmia
Congestive heart failure or evidence for left ventricle (LV) dysfunction, complicated MI
Obstructive aortic outflow disorder (asymmetric septal hypertrophy, aortic stenosis)
Uncontrolled hypertension
Pericardial tumors or cysts
Cardiac vegetations or endocarditis
Acute pericarditis

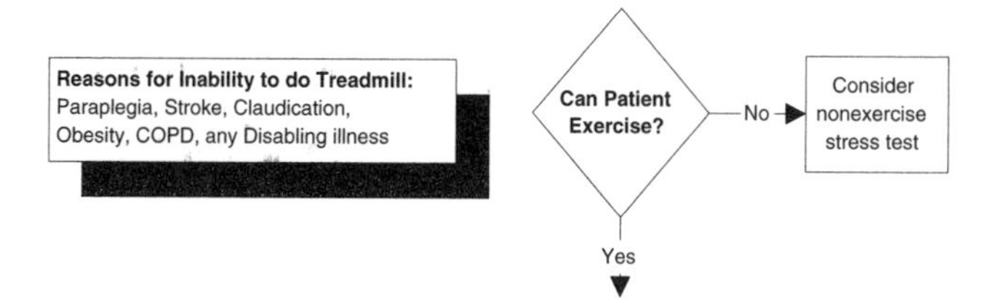

INABILITY TO EXERCISE

History and examination findings reveal which patients are unable to exercise on the treadmill. Listed below are conditions that affect exercise performance, along with selected assessment techniques to evaluate the extent of the condition:

1. **Obesity:** Calculate body mass index (wt/ht^2 in kg and meters); values greater than 32 are considered indicative of obesity.
2. **Pulmonary disease:** physical examination (percussion, diaphragmatic level and movement, and timed forced expiration without pursued lips), pulmonary function test.
3. **Neurologic disease:** Complete neurologic examination for deficits (i.e., paraplegia, stroke).
4. **Orthopedic disability:** Have patient walk to assess gait.
5. **Claudication:** Assess decreased peripheral pulses, signs of vascular insufficiency, bruits.
6. **Disabling illness or secondary weakness:** Perform review of symptoms.
7. **Instability, vertigo:** Assess gait, check postural blood pressures, check for nystagmus.

Pharmacologic Stress Tests

If patients have a negative test, possibly due to inadequate stress (particularly because of an inadequate heart rate and systolic blood pressure [double product] since these functions determine myocardial oxygen demand), or if the patient cannot exercise because of one or more of the above reasons, a pharmacologic stress test should be considered.

The two most commonly used pharmacologic tests are **dipyridamole** (Persantine) (or adenosine) perfusion imaging (using thallium or isonitriles tagged with technetium) and **dobutamine** (or arbutamine) echocardiography. These relatively new tests appear to have excellent characteristics for diagnosing coronary disease and estimating its severity. They are indicated for patients who cannot exercise due to peripheral vascular disease or to neurologic or muscular disease or disability due to other disease. They are also indicated in patients judged to give an inadequate effort during a standard exercise test.

Dipyridamole operates by releasing adenosine, which steals blood flow in the coronary circulation by dilating normal coronary arteries without affecting obstructive lesions. Dobutamine and other chronotropic agents increase heart rate and myocardial oxygen demand and bring out wall motion abnormalities that can be visualized by the echocardiogram. This can also be accomplished by echocardiography in ambulatory patients after treadmill exercise; however, its diagnostic characteristics have not been determined.

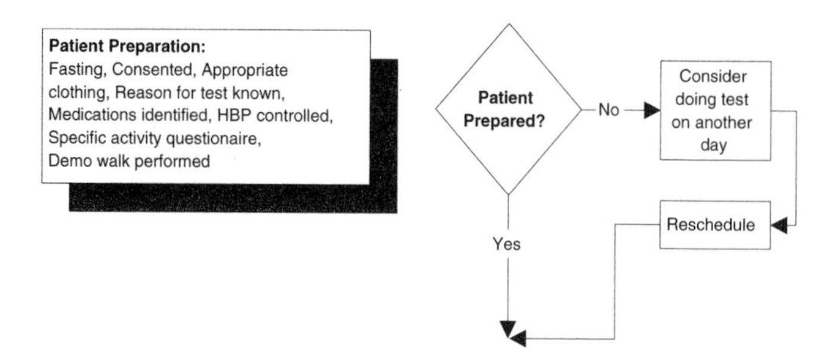

INCOMPLETE PATIENT PREPARATION

Preparation instruction should be given to the patient the day the test is scheduled.

Time of Scheduling Test

The instructions at the time of scheduling should include the following:

1. Do not eat or smoke within 2 to 3 hours of testing. Alcohol and caffeinated drinks should not be ingested for 3 hours prior to testing.
2. Wear comfortable clothing and shoes.
3. Bring prescribed, labeled medication bottles to the testing laboratory so all medications can be accurately recorded. Because of the life-threatening rebound phenomena associated with beta-blocker cessation, these medications should not be stopped routinely prior to testing. However, if testing is performed for diagnostic purposes, they can be gradually stopped if a physician or nurse carefully supervises the tapering-off process.

Time of Test

During the actual time of the test, the following patient-related items should be completed:

1. The reason that the referring physician had for requesting the test should be clearly apparent. If the reason is not apparent, the referring physician should be contacted.
2. A 12-lead electrocardiogram should be obtained in both the supine and standing positions, and the supine ECG compared with any previous supine ECG. The latter is an important rule, particularly in patients with known

heart disease, since an abnormality may prohibit testing. On occasion, a patient referred for an exercise test will instead be admitted to the coronary care unit. The standing ECG is important to detect individuals in whom ST depression has developed below the isoelectric line on standing. If such ST depression occurs, the ST level noted in the standing position is the level from which further ST depression should be measured rather than the isoelectric PQ point. If this is not done, tests on such individuals are likely to result in false positives.

3. There should be careful explanation of why the test is being performed, of the testing procedure including its risks and possible complications, and of how the test is performed. The latter explanation should include the following:

   A demonstration of getting on and off as well as walking on the treadmill
   Instructing the patient that he or she can hold onto the handrails initially, but later on should use the rails only for balance
   Lessening of the test's emotional stress by explaining to the patient that he or she is in charge of the test, which will be stopped when they ask that it be stopped, that this experience will not be the worst of the day, and that the testing is not a pass/fail situation
   That it is better to allow the operators to stop the test rather than for the patient to jump off

4. There should be written or verbal communication or both with the patient and any significant other to explain the exercise testing procedure, risk, and results.
5. If the patient has a known history of hypertension, the blood pressure should be controlled for at least the last 1 to 2 weeks.
6. It is advisable for a staff member to perform a demonstration walk for the patient prior to exercise testing.

Failure to complete the above items may alter the interpretation of results or require rescheduling of the test.

Methodologic Considerations

A strict approach to methodology and technical detail is critical to obtaining accurate and reproducible results from any test.

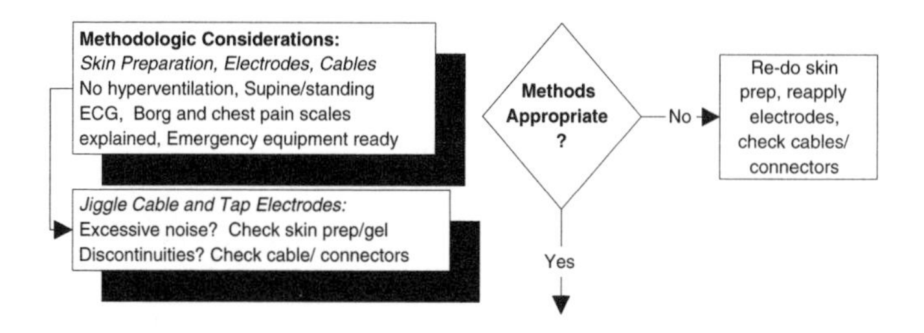

TEN STEPS TO A RELIABLE TEST

The following steps must be observed to assure the test is performed properly.

1. Safety Precautions and Risks

Everything necessary for cardiopulmonary resuscitation must be available, and regular drills should be performed to ascertain that both personnel and equipment are ready for a cardiac emergency. Surveys of clinical exercise facilities[1] have demonstrated exercise testing to be a safe procedure, with approximately one death and five nonfatal complications per 10,000 tests. A recent report[2] of more than 70,000 exercise tests conducted over a 16-year period revealed a complication rate of 0.8 per 10,000 tests.

2. Skin Preparation

Proper skin preparation is essential for the performance of an exercise test. During exercise, because noise increases with the square of resistance, it is extremely important to lower the resistance at the skin-electrode interface, thereby improving the signal-to-noise ratio. It is often difficult for technicians to prepare the skin properly consistently because of patient discomfort and minor skin irritation with increased abrasive measures. These measures are critical because the patient cannot be continuously monitored with artifact present, and this can be a dangerous situation.

The general areas for electrode placement are shaved (if covered with hair) and cleansed with an alcohol-saturated gauze pad. Then, the exact areas for electrode application are marked with a felt-tip pen. The marks serve as a guide for removal of the superficial layer of skin. The superficial layer of skin is removed either with a hand-held drill or by light abrasion with fine-grain emery paper or 3-M electrode paper. Skin resistance should be reduced to 5,000 ohms or less, which can be verified prior to the exercise test with an inexpensive AC impedance meter driven at 10 Hertz.

3. Electrodes and Cables

Cables develop continuity problems with use over time and require replacement rather than repair. Replacement is often necessary after extensive use. Careful skin preparation and attention to the electrode-cable interface are necessary regardless of the sophistication or expense of the ECG recording device.

4. Electrode Placement

1. The electrodes are placed using anatomic landmarks that are found with the patient supine.
2. In some individuals with loose skin, a considerable shift of electrode positions can occur when they assume an upright position.
3. Be sure that V5 and V6 are on a straight line from V4 and do not curve up the rib interspaces. V3 can only be located after V2 and V4 are placed. V3 is half-way between them. V1 and V2 are parasternal in the fourth left and right intercostal spaces.
4. Because a 12-lead ECG cannot be obtained accurately during exercise with electrodes placed on the wrists and ankles, the electrodes are placed at the base of the limbs for exercise testing.
5. The left leg reference for Einthoven's triangle is placed below the umbilicus, and the right leg ground electrode is best placed low on the back over the spine. These points for electrode placement are illustrated in Fig. 8-1.
6. Distortion of the pretest ECG can be kept to a minimum by keeping the arm electrodes off the chest, placing them on the shoulders, and recording the baseline ECG supine. In this situation, the modified exercise limb lead placement can serve as the reference resting ECG prior to an exercise test.[3]
7. Because most meaningful ST depression occurs in the lateral leads (V4, 5, 6) when the resting ECG is normal,

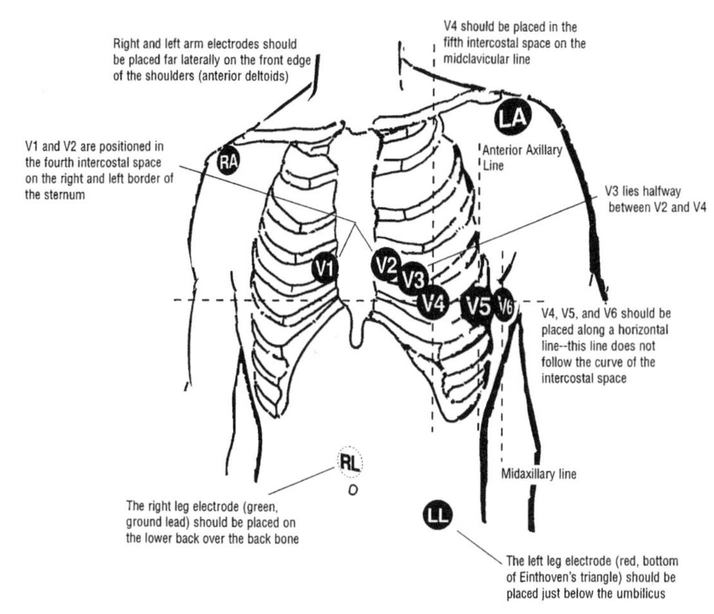

Fig. 8-1. The modified Exercise 12-lead electrode placement.

other leads are only essential in patients with prior MI in whom ECG are distorted by Q waves, in those with a history consistent with coronary spasm or variant angina, or in those in whom exercise-induced arrhythmias are of an uncertain type.

5. ECG Recording

Signal averaging can actually distort the ECG signal. These computerized techniques are attractive because they can produce a clean tracing in spite of noise, even that due to poor skin preparation. The clean-looking ECG signal produced may not be a true representation of the actual wave form and, in fact, may be dangerously misleading.

Consider the raw ECG data first and then use the averages and filtered data to aid interpretation if no distortion is obvious.

6. Borg Scale

1. Rather than using heart rate as the only means to determine clinically the intensity of exercise, it is preferable to consider also the 6 to 20 Borg scale (Fig. 8-2).[4]
2. The 6 to 20 scale was developed by noting that young men could approximate their exercise heart rate if a

6	
7	Very, very light
8	
9	Very light
10	
11	Fairly light
12	
13	Somewhat hard
14	
15	Hard
16	
17	Very hard
18	
19	Very, very hard
20	

Fig. 8-2. The linear 6-to-20 Borg scale of perceived exertion or pain.

scale ranging from 60 to 200 was aligned with labels of very, very light for 60 to very, very hard for 200. One zero was dropped, and the scale was used for all ages.

3. In determining whether an effort is maximal, the Borg scale response should be considered along with age predictions of maximal heart rate and VO_2 and patient appearance.

7. Chest Pain Scale

The 1-to-4 chest pain scale should be used. Care should be taken to see that the pain is evaluated for angina qualities, and it should be specified whether this is the major reason for stopping the test.

8. Hyperventilation *(Do Not Perform!)*

Hyperventilation should not be performed prior to testing. Subjects both with and without disease may or may not exhibit ST-segment changes with hyperventilation; this procedure is no longer considered valuable for identifying false-positive responders.

9. Orthostatic Stress

A standing ECG and BP should always be obtained prior to testing. This will identify patients with orthostatic hypotension and those who exhibit ST-segment depression with standing. The ST response to exercise should be taken from the level observed if it is below the isoelectric PQ point.

10. Blood Pressure Measurement
None of the automated BP devices are reliable for accurate measurements. They are particularly problematic with regard to identifying exertional hypotension. Blood pressure should be taken using a stethoscope manually.

CONCLUSION

This methodologic list (Steps 1–10) should be followed for every exercise test performed to assure accurate and safe data collection.

REFERENCES

1. Rochmis P, Blackburn H. Exercise tests: A survey of procedures, safety, and litigation experience in approximately 170,000 tests. *JAMA* 217:1061–1066, 1971.
2. Gibbons L, Blair SN, Kohl HW, Cooper K. The safety of maximal exercise testing. *Circulation* 80:846–852, 1989.
3. Gamble P, McManus H, Jensen D, Froelicher VF. A comparison of the standard 12-lead electrocardiogram to exercise electrode placements. *Chest* 85:616–622, 1984.
4. Borg G. Perceived exertion as an indicator of somatic stress. *Scand J Rehabil Med* 23:92–93, 1970.

Choosing the Protocol

GENERAL INFORMATION

Dynamic exercise is defined as rhythmic muscular activity resulting in movement, and initiates a more appropriate increase in cardiac output and oxygen exchange than does isometric exercise. Because a delivered workload can be accurately calibrated and the physiologic response easily measured, dynamic exercise is preferred for clinical testing. Although bicycling is a dynamic exercise, most individuals perform more work on a treadmill because a greater muscle mass is involved and most subjects are more familiar with walking than cycling. Maximal heart rate is usually about the same with both devices, but VO_2 max is about 10% higher with a treadmill.

The most common protocols, their stages, and the predicted oxygen cost of each stage are illustrated in Chapter 3 (see Fig. 3-1). Once the most commonly used protocol, the Bruce protocol uses relatively large and unequal increments in work every 3 minutes. Large and uneven work increments such as these have been shown to result in an overestimation of exercise capacity. Currently, protocols with smaller and more equal increments are more often used.

Rather than using the same protocol for every patient, the exercise protocol should be individualized. The optimal test duration is from 8 to 12 minutes, and protocol workloads should be adjusted to permit this duration.[1,2] Ramp testing and other protocols that use small increments permit a more accurate estimation of exercise capacity, particularly when individualized for every patient to yield a targeted test duration by the use of an activity questionnaire.

QUESTIONNAIRES ESTIMATING EXERCISE CAPACITY

Key to ramp testing is that the maximal work capacity be accurately predicted and used as the target for maximal exercise. If a previous test is not available, an accurate questionnaire is critical to setting a ramp and individualizing a test. It is much better to use the Duke Activity Scale (Table 9-1), the VAMC questionnaire (Fig. 9-1), or to question a patient regarding usual activities that have a known METS cost[3] than to use functional class.

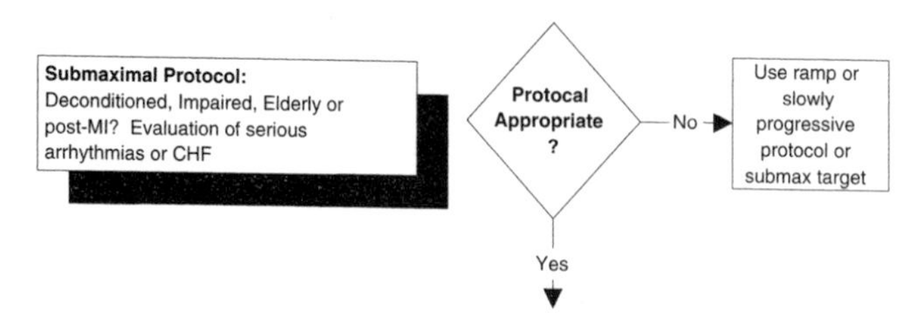

HOW TO CHOOSE THE CORRECT PROTOCOL

Patients referred to the exercise laboratory may perform a maximum or submaximum protocol, depending on past medical history and current symptoms.

Maximum Protocol

1. The exercise protocol should be targeted for the patient rather than the converse.
2. Rapidly paced protocols may be suited to screening younger and/or active individuals (i.e., Bruce, Ellestad), whereas more moderate ones are adapted to older and/or deconditioned patients (i.e., Naughton, Balke-Ware, U.S. Air Force School of Aerospace Medicine).
3. Treadmill speed should be targeted to the individual's capabilities.

Table 9-1. The Duke Activity Scale Index (DASI)

Activity	*Weight*
Can you	
1. Take care of yourself (i.e., eating, dressing, bathing, using the toilet)?	2.75
2. Walk indoors, such as around your house?	1.75
3. Walk a block or two on level ground?	2.75
4. Climb a flight of stairs or walk up a hill?	5.50
5. Run a short distance?	8.00
6. Do light work around the house like dusting or washing dishes?	2.70
7. Do moderate work around the house like vacuuming, sweeping floors, or carrying in groceries?	3.50
8. Do heavy work around the house like scrubbing floors or lifting or moving heavy furniture?	8.00
9. Do yard work like raking leaves, weeding, or pushing a power mower?	4.50
10. Have sexual relations?	5.25
11. Participate in moderate recreational activities such as golf, bowling, dancing, or doubles tennis or throw a basketball or football?	6.00
12. Participate in strenuous sports such as swimming, singles tennis, football, basketball, or sking?	7.50

Notes: The index equals the sum of weights for "yes" replies.
Vo_2 (oxygen uptake) = 0.43 × DASI + 9.6.

Draw one line below the activities you are able to do routinely with minimal or no symptoms such as shortness of breath, chest discomfort, fatigue.

1 MET:
Eating, getting dressed, working at a desk

2 METS:
Taking a shower
Walking down eight steps

3 METS:
Walking slowly on a flat surface for 1 or 2 blocks
Doing a **moderate** amount of work around the house such as vacuuming, sweeping the floors, or carrying groceries

4 METS:
Doing light yard work (i.e., raking leaves, weeding, or pushing a power mower)
Painting or doing light carpentry

5 METS:
Walking briskly (i.e., 4 mi/hr)
Dancing, washing the car

6 METS:
Playing nine holes of golf carrying your own clubs
Doing heavy carpentry or mowing lawn with a push mower

7 METS:
Performing heavy outdoor work (i.e., digging, spading soil)
Playing tennis (singles), carrying 60 pounds

8 METS:
Moving heavy furniture
Jogging slowly, climbing stairs quickly, carrying 20 pounds upstairs

9 METS:
Bicycling at a moderate pace, sawing wood, jumping rope (slowly)

10 METS:
Swimming briskly, bicycling up a hill, walking briskly uphill, jogging 6 mi/hr

11 METS:
Skiing cross-country
Playing basketball (full court)

12 METS:
Running briskly and continuously (level ground, 8-min miles)

13 METS:
Doing any competitive activity, including those that involve intermittent sprinting
Running competitively, rowing, backpacking

Fig. 9-1. The VA questionnaire and activity classification.

4. Even steps in workload should be used, and total time should be 8 to 10 minutes.
5. METS, not minutes, should be reported.
6. A ramp protocol, or protocols with small, even steps permit more accurate estimations of aerobic exercise capacity.

Submaximum Protocol

1. The postmyocardial infarction (MI) or pulmonary patient and deconditioned or impaired, elderly patient may need a slowly progressive protocol or a submaximal MET target level.
2. Submaximal end points used for predischarge testing after an MI include a heart rate from 110 to 120 and a Borg scale of 16 to 17.

REFERENCES

1. Panza JA, Quyyumi AA, Diodati JG, Callaham TS, Epstein SE. Prediction of the frequency and duration of ambulatory myocardial ischemia in patients with stable coronary artery disease by determination of the ischemic threshold from exercise testing: Importance of the exercise protocol. *J Am Coll Cardiol* 17:657–663, 1991.
2. Redwood DR, Rosing DR, Goldstein RE, Beiser GD, Epstein SE. Importance of the design of an exercise protocol in the evaluation of patients with angina pectoris. *Circulation* 43:618–628, 1971.
3. Hlatky M, Boineau R, Higgenbotham M, Lee K, Mark D, Califf R, Cobb F, Prior D. A bried, self-administered questionnaire to determine functional capacity (The Duke Activity Status Index). *Am J Cardiol* 64:651–654, 1989.

Performing the Test

STARTING THE TEST

The patient should be allowed to hold on at first and even be stabilized by the doctor until he or she is accustomed to treadmill walking. If the patient does not appear able to perform the initial level of exercise, alterations should be made to make the test easier. It should be possible to advance or set back the workload of a stage at any point during testing.

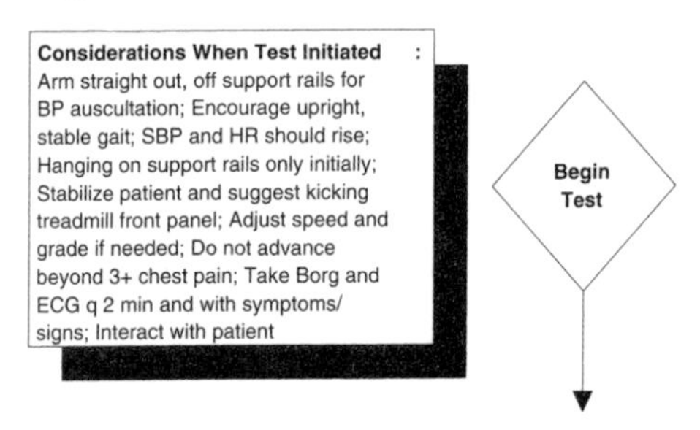

Normal Response

Heart rate (HR) and systolic blood pressure (SBP) should gradually rise throughout the test with the greatest values occurring at peak exercise.

Techniques During Testing

Blood Pressure Measurement

1. The patient's arm should be free of the hand rails such that noise is not transmitted up the arm.
2. It is sometimes helpful to mark the brachial artery.
3. If SBP appears to be slowly increasing or decreasing, it should be taken again immediately.
4. If a drop in SBP of 20 mm Hg or more occurs after a rise or if it drops below the value obtained in the standing position prior to testing, the test should be stopped in patients with congestive heart failure, myocardial damage, or a prior myocardial infarction. The test should also be stopped in those patients who are exhibiting signs/symptoms of ischemia or arrhythmias.
5. An increase in SBP to 260 mm Hg or an increase in diastolic blood pressure to 115 mm Hg is also a relative indication to stop the test.
6. Record blood pressure at least every 2 minutes and when any signs or symptoms occur.

ECG Recording Instrumentation

1. While notched 60-Hz filters are fine, do not turn on the filters that reject all frequencies greater than 59 Hz. Make sure the frequency response and paper speed are appropriate.
2. Consider the raw ECG data first (observe three consecutive, consistent complexes and then use the computer averages and measurements to aid interpretation if no distortion is obvious).

The Treadmill

1. The treadmill should have front and side rails for patients to use to steady themselves, and some patients may benefit from the helping hand of the person administering the test.
2. Do not allow anyone to stand on the treadmill belt before it is turned on. A sudden start could cause injury.
3. An emergency stop button should be readily available to the staff only.
4. A small platform or stepping area at the level of the belt is advisable such that the patient can start the test by "pedaling" the belt with one foot prior to stepping onto it.
5. Patients should not grasp the front or side rails as this decreases the work performed and oxygen uptake, which increases exercise time, resulting in an overestimation of exercise capacity. Gripping the handrails also increases ECG muscle artifact.
6. It can be helpful to have patients take their hands off the rails, close their fists, and extend one finger to touch the rails to maintain balance while walking, after they are accustomed to the treadmill.
7. Some patients may require a few moments to feel comfortable enough to let go of the handrails, but strongly discourage grasping the handrails after the first minute of exercise.

Interaction with the Patient

1. Converse with the patient to decrease anxiety and assess symptoms.
2. Touch skin to assess for diaphoresis, coolness, and adequacy of perfusion.
3. Request the Borg scale every 2 minutes and specifically ask about the occurrence of chest pain. This is the best opportunity to determine if the patient really has angina since he or she is actually experiencing the sensation at the time.

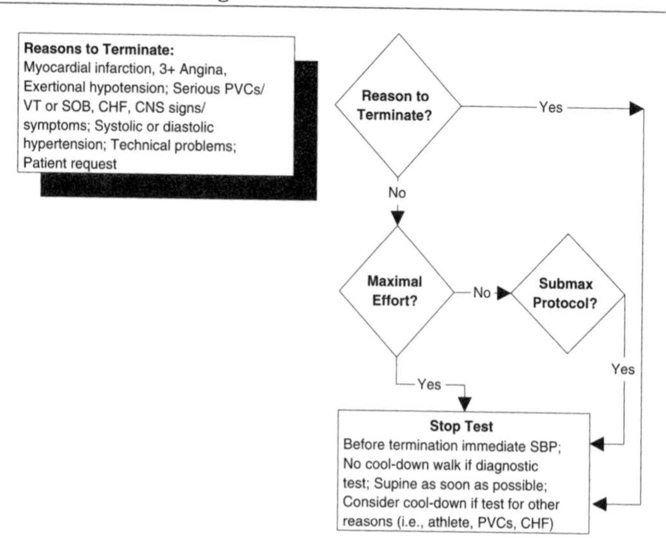

TEST TERMINATION

Absolute Reasons or Indications to Terminate

1. Acute myocardial infarction.
2. Severe angina: Chest pain score of 4 out of 4.
3. Exertional hypotension: If a drop in SBP of 20 mm Hg or more occurs or if it drops below the value obtained in the standing position prior to testing, the test should be stopped in patients with congestive heart failure or a prior myocardial infarction, or in those who are exhibiting signs/symptoms of ischemia.
4. Serious arrhythmias: Ventricular tachycardia, third degree heart block.
5. Poor perfusion as judged by skin temperature and cyanosis.
6. Neurologic signs: Confusion, lightheadedness, vertigo, headache.
7. Technical problems: Inability to interpret the ECG pattern, any malfunction of the recording or monitoring device, inability to measure the SBP.
8. Patient's request.

Relative Reasons or Indications to Terminate

The following indications may be superseded if done so for good clinical reasons:

1. More than 3 mm ST shift.
2. Increasing chest pain: Chest pain score of 3.
3. Pronounced fatigue and shortness of breath.

4. Wheezing.
5. Leg pain or claudication.
6. An increase in SBP to 260 mm Hg or an increase in diastolic blood pressure to 115 mm Hg can be an indication to stop the test.
7. Less serious arrhythmia.
8. Bundle branch block or another rate-dependent intraventricular conduction defect that presents similarly to ventricular tachycardia.

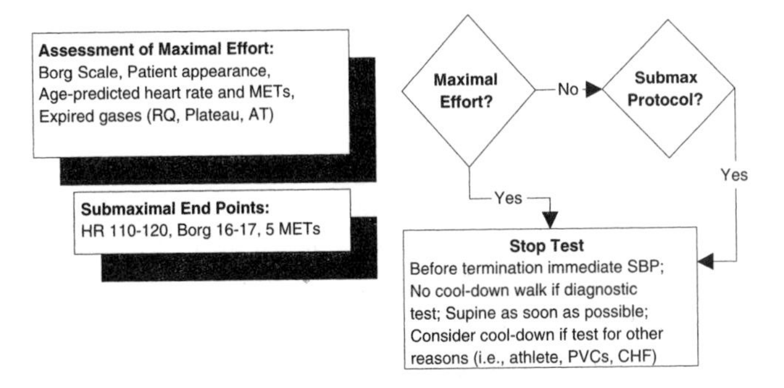

Assessment of Maximal Effort

Because no single marker of effort is usually specifically indicative of a maximal effort, it is best to consider multiple responses:

1. Borg scale of 17 or greater.
2. Signs of fatigue, profound shortness of breath, or exhaustion.
3. Age-predicted maximal heart rate particularly when a population specific regression equation is used.
4. METS level reached compared with the age-predicted METS value.
5. Expired gas measurements including respiratory quotient greater than 1.1 and a plateau of $\dot{V}O_2$.
6. Double product should exceed 25,000.

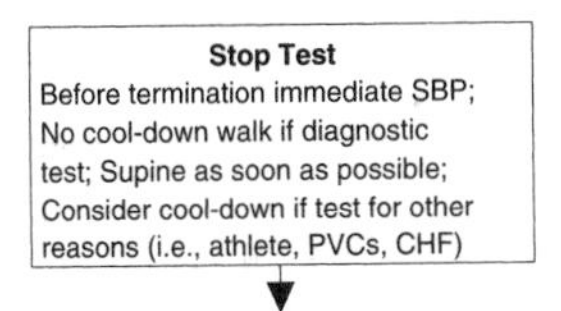

Maximal Exercise or Termination Point

1. A maximum heart rate, blood pressure, and ECG should be taken immediately before the exercise test

has been terminated. These values represent the patient's maximum hemodynamic and ECG response.

2. Usually, ECG changes occurring within 30 seconds of stopping are considered exercise responses, and only the measurements made later are considered as part of recovery.

Recovery Methods:
NTG can cause hypotension so do not administer; Monitor ECG for at least 5 min or until changes stabilize; Always record 3 min post-exercise ECG since it is very important; Sit patient up if Severe Ischemia, CHF, or PVCs occur

Recovery
Supine, monitor SBP, symptoms and ECG each minute for 5 min; Emergency procedures as needed; If new ST depression occurs, monitor ECG until the changes stabilize

RECOVERY/POSTEXERCISE PERIOD

1. If the patient performs a cool-down walk after the test, it can delay or eliminate the appearance of ST segment depression.[1]
2. If maximal sensitivity for diagnosing coronary artery disease is to be achieved with an exercise test, patients should be supine during the postexercise period.
3. It is advisable to record about 10 seconds of electrocardiographic data while the patient is standing motionless, but still experiencing near maximal heart rate, and then have them lie down. Some patients must be allowed to lie down immediately to avoid hypotension due to peripheral pooling.
4. According to the law of La Place, the increase in venous return, and thus ventricular volume, in the supine position increases myocardial oxygen demand.[2]
5. The supine position after exercise is not so important when the test is not being performed for diagnostic purposes. When testing is not performed for diagnostic purposes, it may be preferable to walk slowly (1.0–1.5 mph) or continue cycling against zero or minimal resistance (0–25 Watts when testing with a cycle ergometer) for several minutes after the test.
6. Patients who cannot tolerate an increase preload, such as cardiomyopathy patients, should sit immediately after exercise.
7. Monitoring should continue for at least 5 minutes after exercise or until changes stabilize.
8. Approximately 85% of patients with abnormal responses will have an abnormal response in the supine position 3 to 5 minutes into recovery only or in addition to other times.

REFERENCES

1. Gutman RA, Alexander ER, Li YB, Bruce R. Delay of ST depression after maximal exercise by walking for two minutes. *Circulation* 42:229–233, 1970.
2. Lachterman B, Lehmann KG, Abrahamson D, Froelicher VF. "Recovery only" ST segment depression and the predictive accuracy of the exercise test. *Ann Intern Med* 112:11–16, 1990.

Add-ons to Standard Exercise ECG Testing

MEASURED EXPIRED GASES

Because of the inaccuracies associated with estimating METS (ventilatory oxygen consumption) from workload (i.e., treadmill speed and grade), measurement of the expired gases is sometimes indicated. Although this requires additional equipment and either a mouthpiece in the patient's mouth or a face mask during exercise, it can be done safely if the patient is taught how to use hand signs for his or her symptoms. Although it is not necessary for all clinical testing, expired gas analysis also permits measurement of other parameters, including respiratory quotient (RQ), efficiency of ventilation, physiologic dead space, plateauing, and ventilatory anaerobic threshold. Anaerobic threshold can also be determined by measuring blood lactate levels during exercise. This measurement is helpful because it determines the comfortable submaximal exercise limit for the performance of daily activities and can be used for setting optimal exercise prescriptions. Whereas serial testing is associated with increases in exercise workload due to habituation or learning, measured METS are stable.

PRECORDIAL WALL MOTION SENSORS

The apex cardiogram, displacement cardiograph (DCG) or kinetocardiogram, and the siesmocardiogram were all devices purported to diagnose coronary artery disease by sensing anterior cardiac wall motion abnormalities. The sensing device is placed on the chest after exercise and left ventricular wall motion assessed indirectly.

ECHOCARDIOGRAMS

The ECG-gated freeze frame echocardiogram can be captured after treadmill exercise and compared with resting recorded images to detect wall motion abnormalities induced by ischemia. The reproducibility and specificity of these abnormalities has yet to be determined. Many patients cannot be studied because of poor echocardiographic imaging characteristics (i.e., smokers, the obese).

RADIONUCLIDE EXERCISE TESTING

Basically there are two types of radionuclide exercise testing currently available: ventricular function testing (using the first pass or computer-averaged [MUGA] methods of observing the passage of technetium-tagged red cells through the heart) and perfusion imaging (using thallium or technetium-tagged isonitriles). They both require intravenous access for injection of a radioactive substance and imaging with a standard gamma camera. The ventricular function is observed during supine cycle ergometry exercise, and in general the ejection fraction should increase in healthy subjects and decline (or exhibit wall motion abnormalities) in patients with ischemia. Various criteria have been tried, but unfortunately the poor specificity of this test makes it unsuitable for most clinical purposes. Because perfusion imaging has test characteristics that exceed the standard exercise ECG, it is the first additional test when the standard exercise test is equivocal or incongruous with other clinical findings or symptoms. It also permits the localization of ischemia to a coronary artery distribution, which is not possible with the standard exercise test. Thallium scintigraphy is rarely indicated as the primary test because the standard exercise test is more convenient and cost-effective. Recently, the addition of three-dimensional imaging (SPECT) has increased the sensitivity but decreased the specificity of the test.

Key Points from Part II

1. Preparing the patient physically and emotionally for testing is necessary.
2. Good skin preparation must cause some discomfort but is necessary to avoid artifact.
3. The use of specific criteria for exclusion from testing and termination, physician interaction with the patient, and availability of appropriate emergency equipment are essential.
4. A brief physical examination is always necessary to rule out significant aortic valve disease and other high-risk cardiac abnormalities.
5. Pretest standard 12-lead ECG are needed in both the supine (for comparison with prior ECG and to interpret infarction patterns) and standing positions (for determination of the ST level at which to compare exercise-induced changes).
6. The changes caused by exercise electrode placement can be kept to a minimum by keeping the arm electrodes off the chest, placing them on the shoulders, and recording the baseline ECG supine. In this situation, the modified exercise limb lead placement of Mason and Likar can serve well as the reference resting ECG prior to an exercise test if recorded supine.
7. The exercise protocol should be progressive with equal increments in speed and grade whenever possible. Smaller, even, and more frequent work increments are preferable to larger, uneven, and less frequent increases, because the former yield a more accurate estimation of exercise capacity.
8. Use METS, not minutes, to report exercise capacity from treadmill performance.
9. Individualize the exercise protocol, rather than use the same protocol for every patient. Because the optimal test duration is from 8 to 12 minutes, the protocol workloads should be adjusted to permit this duration.
10. Because ramp testing uses small increments, it permits a more accurate estimation of exercise capacity, and can be individualized for every patient to yield a targeted test duration.

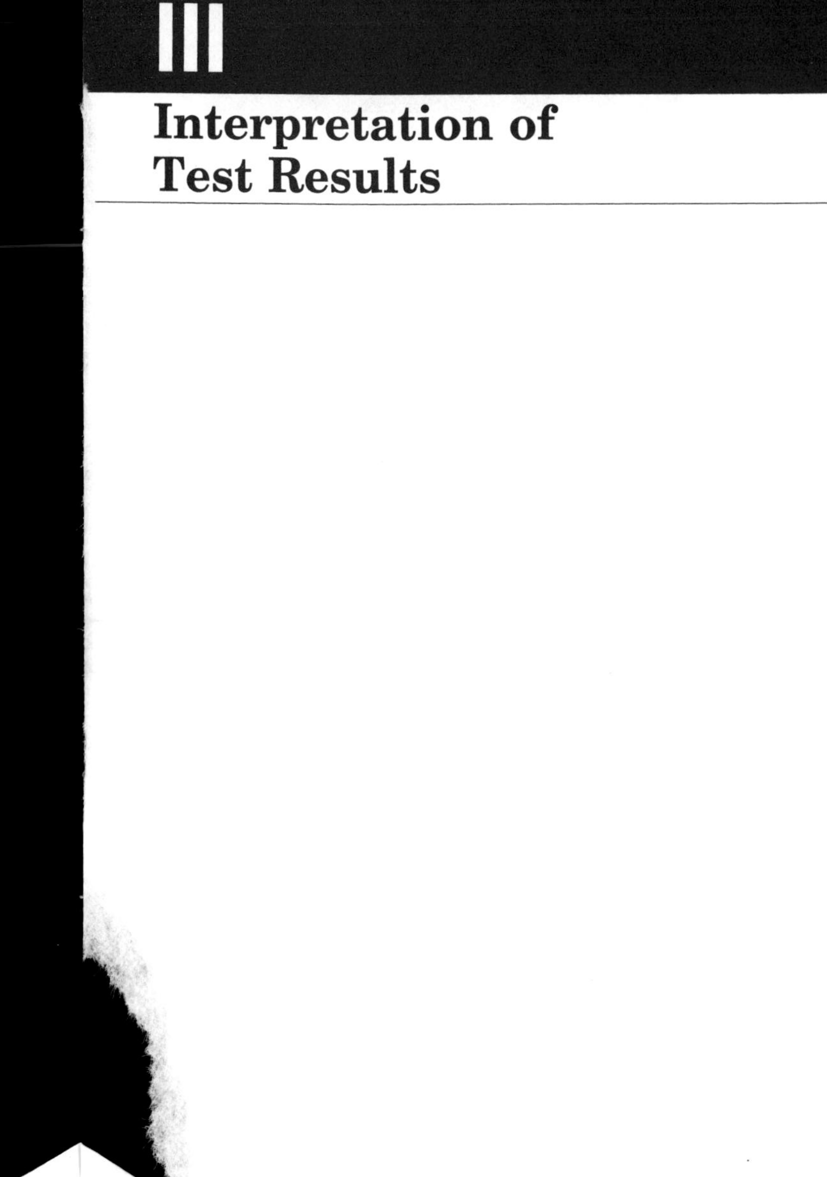

III

Interpretation of Test Results

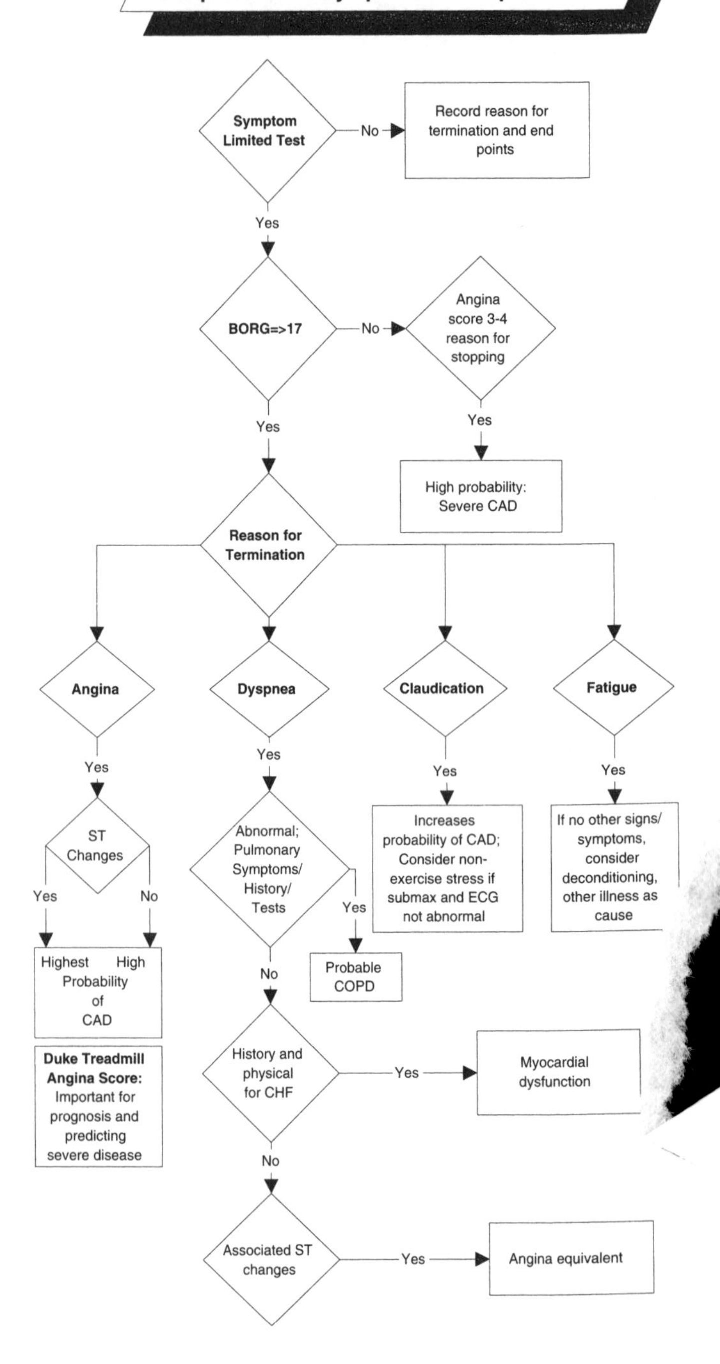

Interpretation of Symptomatic Responses
Symptom Limited Test
No
Record reason for termination and end points
Yes
BORG=>17
No
Angina score 3-4 reason for stopping
Yes
High probability: Severe CAD
Yes
Reason for Termination
Angina
Dyspnea
Claudication
Fatigue
Yes
ST Changes
Yes
No
Highest High Probability of CAD
Duke Treadmill Angina Score: Important for prognosis and predicting severe disease
Yes
Abnormal; Pulmonary Symptoms/ History/ Tests
Yes
Probable COPD
No
History and physical for CHF
Yes
Myocardial dysfunction
No
Associated ST changes
Yes
Angina equivalent
Yes
Increases probability of CAD; Consider non-exercise stress if submax and ECG not abnormal
Yes
If no other signs/ symptoms, consider deconditioning, other illness as cause

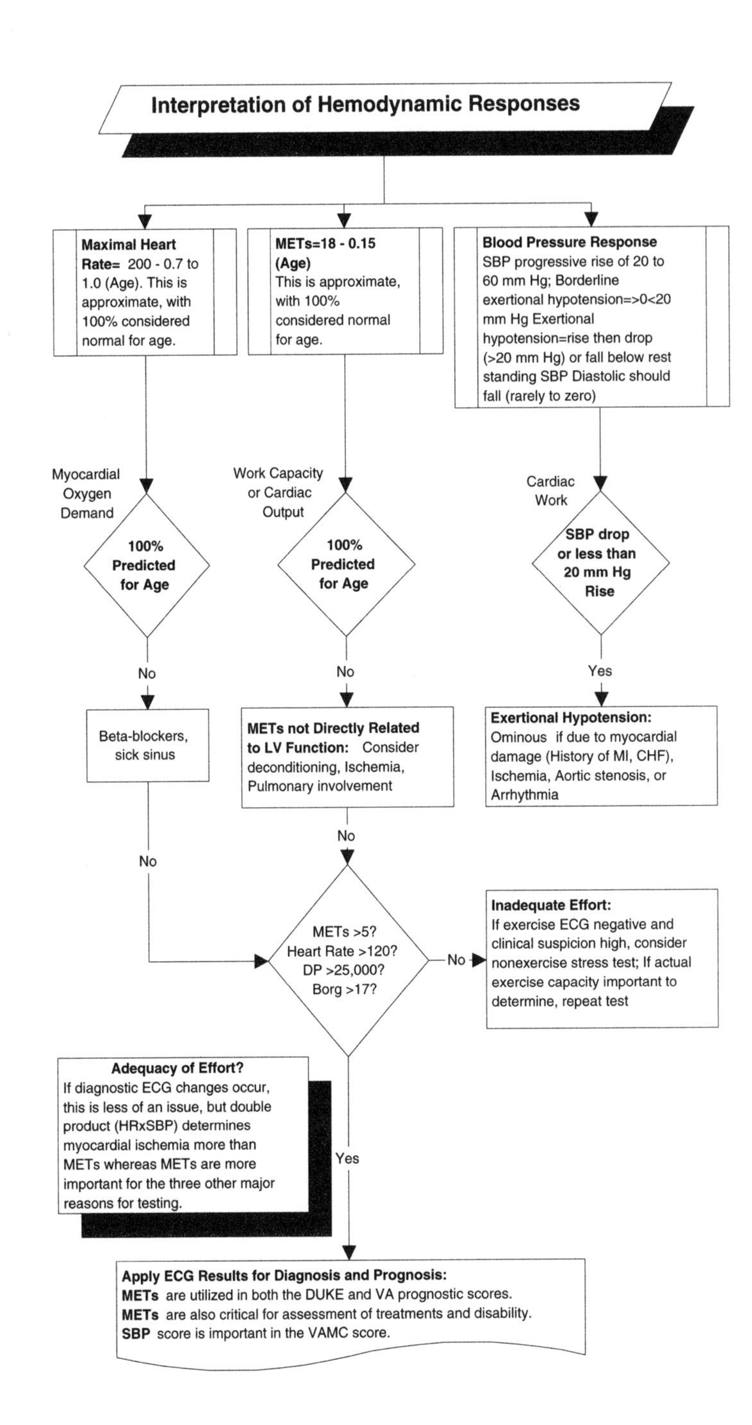

Interpretation of Hemodynamic Responses
Maximal Heart Rate= 200 - 0.7 to 1.0 (Age). This is approximate, with 100% considered normal for age.
METs=18 - 0.15 (Age) This is approximate, with 100% considered normal for age.
Blood Pressure Response SBP progressive rise of 20 to 60 mm Hg; Borderline exertional hypotension=>0<20 mm Hg Exertional hypotension=rise then drop (>20 mm Hg) or fall below rest standing SBP Diastolic should fall (rarely to zero)
Myocardial Oxygen Demand
100% Predicted for Age
Work Capacity or Cardiac Output
100% Predicted for Age
Cardiac Work
SBP drop or less than 20 mm Hg Rise
No
No
Yes
Beta-blockers, sick sinus
METs not Directly Related to LV Function: Consider deconditioning, Ischemia, Pulmonary involvement
Exertional Hypotension: Ominous if due to myocardial damage (History of MI, CHF), Ischemia, Aortic stenosis, or Arrhythmia
No
No
METs >5? Heart Rate >120? DP >25,000? Borg >17?
No
Inadequate Effort: If exercise ECG negative and clinical suspicion high, consider nonexercise stress test; If actual exercise capacity important to determine, repeat test
Adequacy of Effort? If diagnostic ECG changes occur, this is less of an issue, but double product (HRxSBP) determines myocardial ischemia more than METs whereas METs are more important for the three other major reasons for testing.
Yes
Apply ECG Results for Diagnosis and Prognosis:
METs are utilized in both the DUKE and VA prognostic scores.
METs are also critical for assessment of treatments and disability.
SBP score is important in the VAMC score.

Interpretation of the Exercise ECG

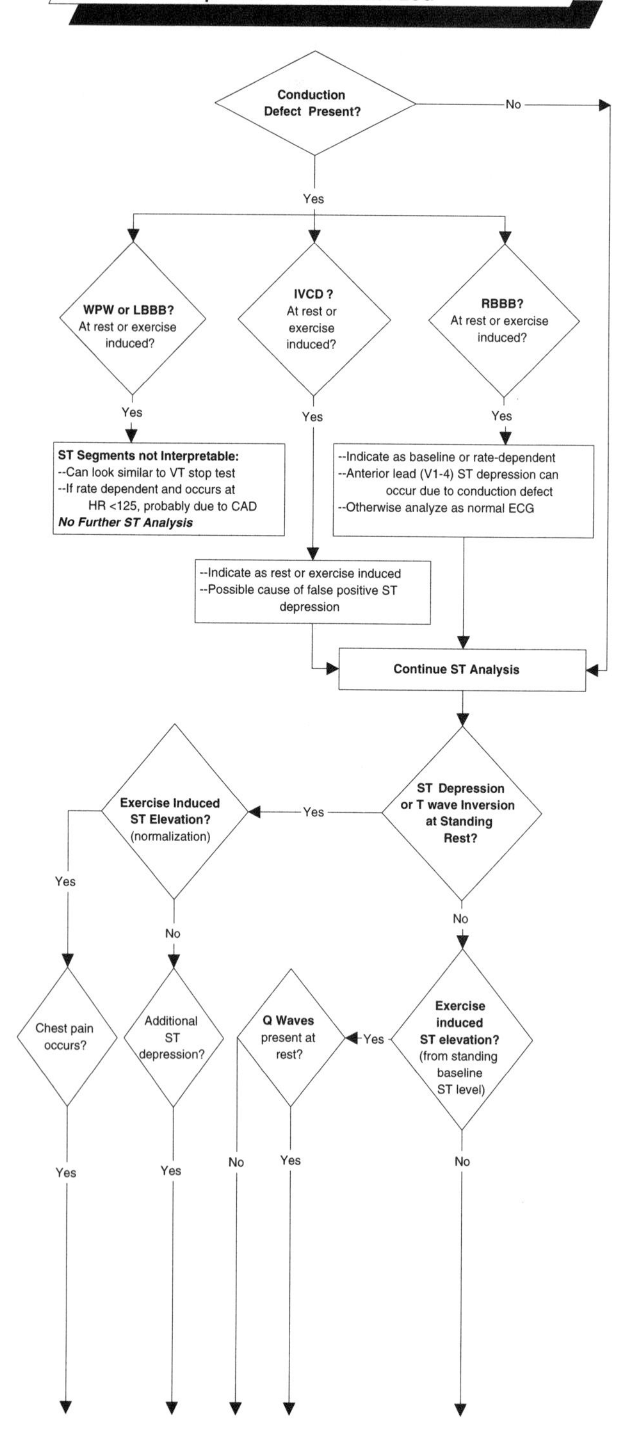

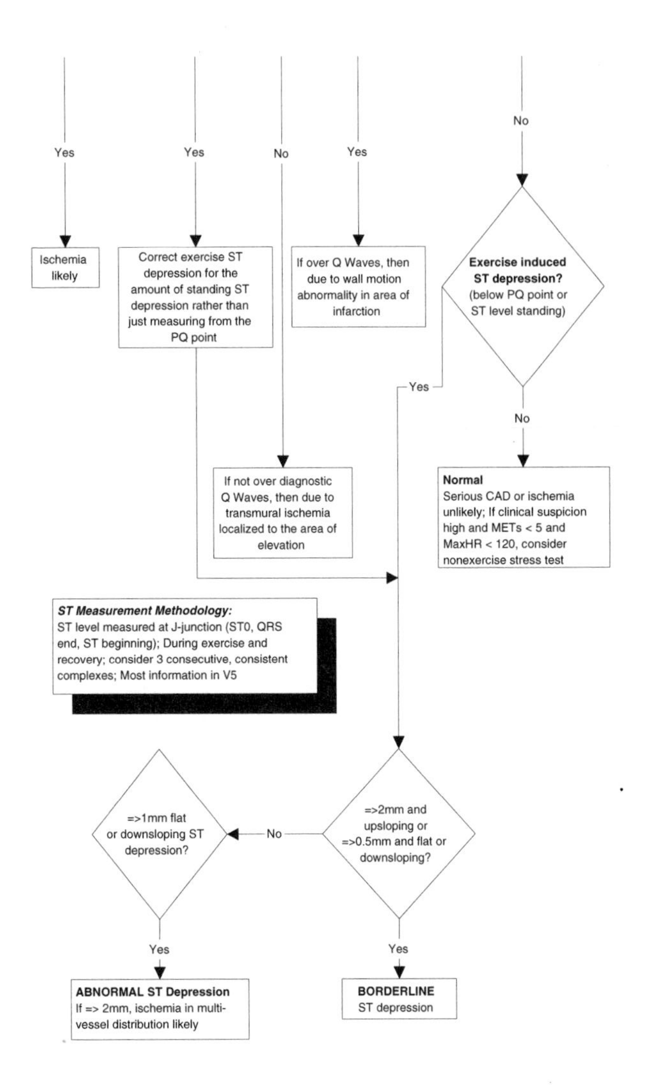
Yes
Yes
No
Yes
No
Ischemia likely
Correct exercise ST depression for the amount of standing ST depression rather than just measuring from the PQ point
If over Q Waves, then due to wall motion abnormality in area of infarction
Exercise induced ST depression? (below PQ point or ST level standing)
Yes
No
If not over diagnostic Q Waves, then due to transmural ischemia localized to the area of elevation
Normal
Serious CAD or ischemia unlikely; If clinical suspicion high and METs < 5 and MaxHR < 120, consider nonexercise stress test
ST Measurement Methodology:
ST level measured at J-junction (ST0, QRS end, ST beginning); During exercise and recovery; consider 3 consecutive, consistent complexes; Most information in V5
=>1mm flat or downsloping ST depression?
No
=>2mm and upsloping or =>0.5mm and flat or downsloping?
Yes
Yes
ABNORMAL ST Depression
If => 2mm, ischemia in multi-vessel distribution likely
BORDERLINE
ST depression

Approach to Interpretation

Interpretation of the exercise test involves analysis of the symptoms/signs, hemodynamic responses, and the ECG. These are systematically reviewed in the chapters that follow. The purpose of this chapter is to outline the recommended thought process for interpreting an exercise test.

First, is there any condition that affected exercise performance or could affect interpretation of the test?

1. **Orthopedic disability:** Was the patient able to walk and was his or her gait impaired?
2. **Pulmonary disease:** Did the physical examination, including timed forced expiration, reveal any abnormalities?
3. **Obesity:** Was the height-weight ratio abnormal?
4. **Neurologic disease:** Were any neurologic deficits present?
5. **Deconditioning:** What was revealed by the questions regarding activities or an activity questionnaire?
6. **Resting ECG abnormality:** Were left and right bundle branch blocks, IVCD, Wolff-Parkinson-White, left ventricular pressure (LVH), diagnostic Q-waves, or ST depression present? (Resting ST depression or LVH will slightly lessen specificity, but sensitivity remains good and the exercise ECG still remains the best first diagnostic test.)
7. **Medications:** Were drugs (particularly beta blockers or digoxin) taken prior to testing?

If any of the above situations affected performance (inadequate effort) or interpretation, causing false, negative test results, a dipyridamole-thallium or dobutamine echo would be a good alternative test. If clinical judgment suggests false-positive test results, would an echo or nuclear add-on to a repeat treadmill test be helpful?

Second, what was the major purpose of the test? If test was performed to diagnose clinically significant coronary disease (i.e., is it present or not present), first determine pretest probability (age, gender, risk factors, but chest pain characteristics dominate).

1. Consider the effects of medications (digoxin affects ST, beta blockers affect heart rate, antihypertensives af-

fect the BP response, antiarrhythmics can be proarrhythmic and affect heart rate).
2. The diagnostic criterion is 1 mm of horizontal or downsloping ST segment shift below the isoelectric PQ point measured at the J-junction. If ST depression is present on the standing, resting ECG, 1 mm additional depression is required.

If the test was performed to determine for prognosis (probability of serious angiographic disease and risk of cardiovascular death) consider the following:

1. The probability of severe angiographic coronary disease is high if 2 mm or more horizontal or downward ST depression occurs. This is especially true at a low workload and low double product persisting into recovery, and if angina is the reason for stopping the test.
2. The risk of cardiovascular death is multifactorial, including clinical assessment (history of congestive heart failure or prior myocardial infarction) and exercise responses (including inadequate systolic blood pressure response or a drop), more than 2-mm ST depression or 1-mm ST elevation in non-Q-wave area, and less than 5 METS maximal exercise capacity.
3. It is better, however, to use the Duke or VAMC prognostic scores, which combine multiple responses and variables resulting in a more accurate prediction of prognosis.

If for evaluation of exercise capacity, be sure that a maximal effort is given, considering safety, and that METS are accurately measured or estimated. Encourage the patient not to hold on and to get to a Borg of 19 or 20.

If for assessment of treatment, establish the baseline for the angina, BP, or arrhythmias that are to be treated and assure that the measurements are reproducible and the methods consistent.

Symptoms and Signs

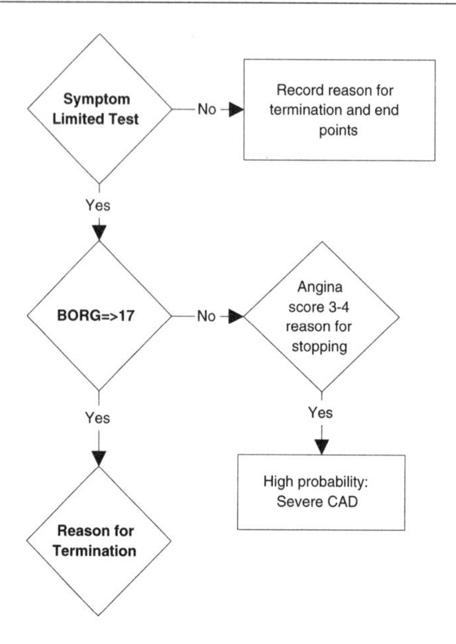

This chapter deals with the symptoms and signs of disease that can be precipitated by the exercise test. They should be carefully elicited and described.

SUBJECTIVE RESPONSES

1. Careful observation of the patient's appearance is necessary for the safe performance of an exercise test and is helpful in the clinical assessment of a patient. Patients who exaggerate their limitations or symptoms, and those unwilling to cooperate, are usually easy to identify.
2. A drop in skin temperature during exercise can indicate an inadequate cardiac output with secondary vasoconstriction, and can be an indication for not encouraging a patient to a higher workload.
3. Neurologic manifestations such as lightheadedness or vertigo can also be indications of an inadequate cardiac output.

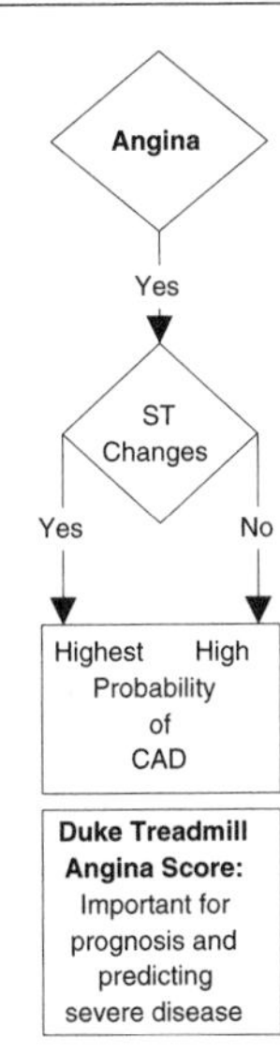

CHEST PAIN

1. The exercise test is the best opportunity to evaluate the characteristics of a patient's exercise-induced chest pain.
2. Explaining their symptoms can be difficult for patients, and they are more concerned with sharp chest pains that are not ischemic or cannot adequately describe their pain.
3. Limitations posed out of the fear of precipitating the pain can be overcome during testing.
4. Multiple types of pain or sensations can be confusing for some patients or in others a stoic disposition will make them reluctant to admit to pain.
5. Careful questioning of the patient and noting of the response to the pain or sensation often result in the most meaningful information obtained during testing.
6. Chest pain must be qualified as noncardiac chest pain, atypical or typical angina pectoris; otherwise the interpretation is inadequate. Also, it should be clear if it is the reason for stopping the test.

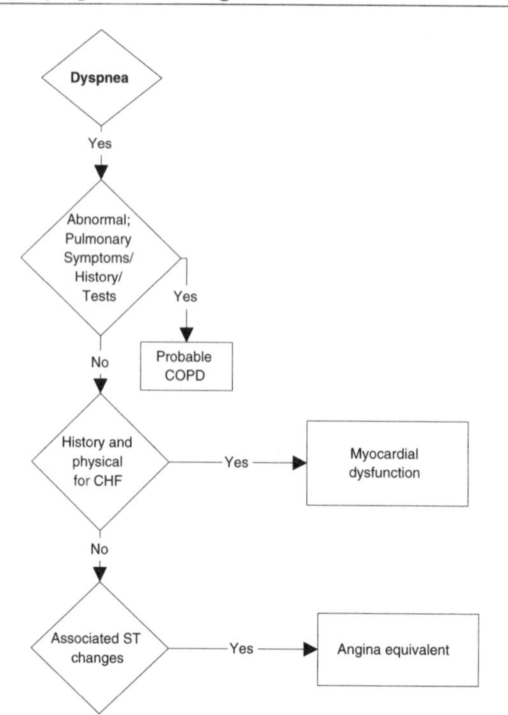

DYSPNEA

1. The cause of dyspnea (i.e., is it due to cardiac disease or lung disease?) can be determined by the exercise test in conjunction with pulmonary function tests. In addition, if dyspnea is due to cardiac disease, whether it is myocardial dysfunction caused by left ventricular damage, diastolic dysfunction, or due to acute ischemia should be determined.
2. Dyspnea can be an anginal equivalent, but the usual indications for this diagnosis are a totally normal resting ECG (i.e., normal resting ejection fraction), normal pulmonary function, and abnormal exercise-induced ST depression.
3. Dyspnea due to pulmonary disease usually occurs in patients with the history, physical examination, and pulmonary function typical of pulmonary disease. Wheezing during the test is another clue to a primary pulmonary cause.
4. Dyspnea of cardiac origin usually occurs in a patient with ECG evidence of myocardial damage, cardiomeg-

aly, and other signs and symptoms of congestive heart failure.

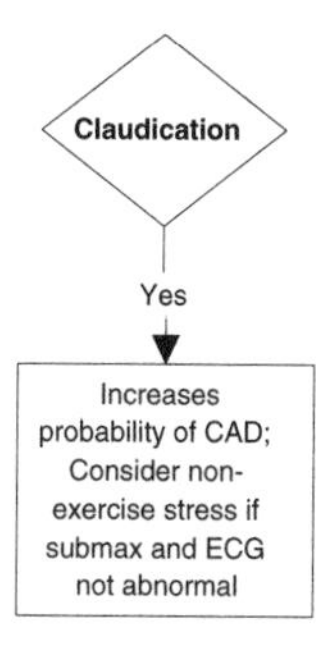

CLAUDICATION

1. Leg or buttocks pain brought on by walking, which is relieved by resting and is not positional (like the similar pain of spinal stenosis) is typical of large vessel vascular disease.
2. When atherosclerosis causes problems in the leg arteries, the probability of obstructive coronary disease is increased.
3. This symptom complex during exercise is usually confirmed by bruits and physical findings of vascular insufficiency such as skin atrophy and loss of hair.

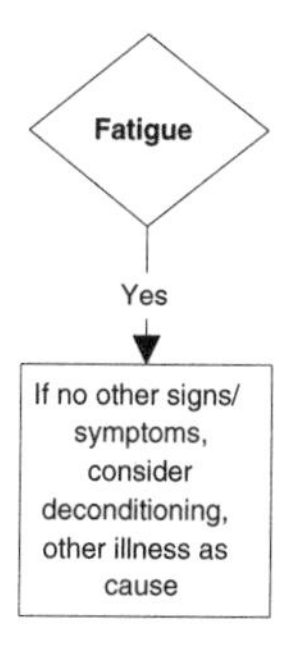

FATIGUE

1. This is a nonspecific response.
2. It usually means that the anaerobic threshold has been exceeded, but if the heart rate and METS are below those expected for age, consider deconditioning, depression, or noncardiac illnesses as the explanation.

PHYSICAL EXAMINATION

1. Findings on physical examination noted after the test can be helpful, but their sensitivity and specificity have not been demonstrated.
2. Gallop sounds, a mitral regurgitant murmur, or a precordial bulge could be due to left ventricular dysfunction.
3. An S3 can sometimes be heard in healthy subjects after exercise, but a new S4 brought out by exercise has been said to be specific for coronary heart disease.
4. Wheezing and sounds of obstructive air way disease could confirm pulmonary disease as the cause of exercise limitation.

Hemodynamic Responses

This chapter deals with the hemodynamic responses to the dynamic exercise performed during the exercise test.

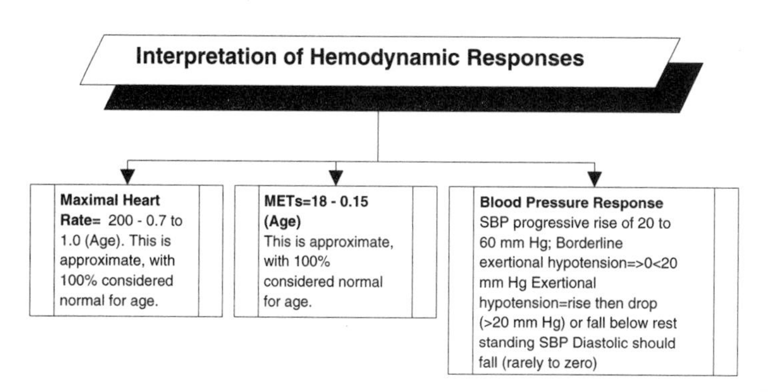

EXERCISE PHYSIOLOGY

1. Total body oxygen uptake and myocardial oxygen uptake are distinct in their determinants and in the way they are measured or estimated (Fig. 14-1).
2. Total body or ventilatory oxygen uptake (VO_2) is the amount of oxygen that is extracted from inspired air as the body works.
3. Myocardial oxygen uptake is the amount of oxygen consumed by the heart muscle.
4. The ST segment response and angina are associated with myocardial ischemia (coronary artery disease), whereas exercise capacity, systolic blood pressure (SBP), and heart rate responses to exercise are determined by myocardial ischemia, myocardial dysfunction, responses in the periphery, or a combination.
5. Exercise-induced ischemia can cause cardiac dysfunction, which results in exercise impairment and an abnormal SBP response. Often it is difficult to separate the effect of ischemia from the effect of left ventricular dysfunction on exercise responses.
6. The severity of ischemia or the amount of myocardium in jeopardy is known clinically to be inversely related to the heart rate, blood pressure, and exercise level achieved. However, neither resting nor exercise ejection fraction (or its change during exercise) correlates well with measured or estimated maximal ventilatory

Myocardial oxygen consumption ≅ Heart rate × systolic blood pressure (determinants include wall tension ≅ left ventricular pressure × volume; contractility; and heart rate)
Ventilatory oxygen consumption (V_{O_2}) ≅ External work performed, or cardiac output × AV_{O_2} difference*

*AV_{O_2} difference is approximately 15% to 17 vol% at maximal exercise; therefore V_{O_2} max is a non-invasive method for estimating cardiac output.

Fig. 14-1. The determinants of the two types of oxygen consumption during exercise.

oxygen uptake even in patients without signs or symptoms of ischemia.[1-3]

MEASURES OF MAXIMAL EFFORT

In clinical practice, assessment of effort should include the following:

The Borg Scale of perceived exertion
Patient appearance and signs and symptoms
Systolic blood pressure response
Double product in excess of 25,000
The percentage of age-predicted maximal heart rate and V_{O_2}

To confirm that a MET value is truly maximal, various objective measurements have been used applying expired gas analysis, scales of perceived exertion, and blood samples:

1. As maximal aerobic capacity is reached, the rate of oxygen consumption may reach a plateau. A decrease or failure to increase oxygen uptake by 150 cc/min with increased workloads is the criterion for the "plateau." However, a plateau is infrequently seen in continuous treadmill protocols and may actually be due to holding onto the handrails, incomplete expired air collection, and methodologic issues such as sampling interval or the equipment used.
2. Respiratory quotient, the ratio of carbon dioxide production to oxygen use, increases in proportion to exercise effort. Values of 1.15 are reached by most individuals at the point of maximal dynamic exercise. However, this varies greatly and requires gas measurements during exercise.
3. Lactic acid levels have also been used (i.e., >7 or 8

mMol), but they also require mixed venous samples and vary greatly among individuals.

4. The Borg scale has been developed to grade subjectively levels of exertion. The linear scale ranges from 6 (very, very light) to 20 (very, very hard), the nonlinear scale ranges from 0 to 10, and both correlate with the percentage of maximal heart rate during exercise.

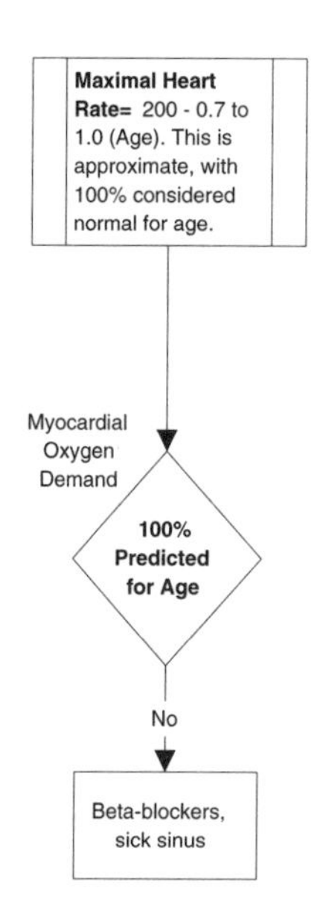

MAXIMAL HEART RATE

Factors Affecting Maximal Heart Rate

1. The heart rate response to exercise is influenced by multiple factors including the following:
   a. Age
   b. Gender
   c. Type of activity
   d. Body size and position
   e. Fitness and bedrest
   f. Cardiac dimensions and mass
   g. Presence of heart disease
   h. Medications
   i. Blood volume
   j. Environment
2. The most important of these factors is age; a decline in maximal heart rate occurs with increasing age. Height,

weight, and even lean body weight apparently do not affect maximal heart rate.[4] Maximal heart rate is determined by intrinsic cardiac changes rather than neural influences.
3. Maximal heart rate is unchanged or may be slightly reduced after exercise training. Resting heart rate is frequently reduced after training, which is due to enhanced parasympathetic tone.
4. Bedrest raises maximal heart rate.[5]
5. Older patients are often restrained by poor muscle tone, pulmonary disease, claudication, orthopedic problems, and other noncardiac causes of limitation. The usual decline in heart rate maximum (HRmax) with age is not as steep in persons who are free of myocardial disease and stay active, but it still occurs.

Chronotropic Incompetence or Heart Rate Impairment
Much of what has been called "chronotropic incompetence" is related to early termination of exercise due to angina pectoris.[6] Nevertheless, there are patients not limited by angina in whom heart rate impairment occurs. These patients also have lower aerobic capacity than age-matched patients with a normal heart rate response.

Estimates of Maximal Heart Rate from Age
1. Although a regression line of 200 − 0.6 (age) is fairly reproducible, the scatter around this line is considerable (i.e., 1 SD = ± 12 bpm). Because such predictions are maximal for some individuals and submaximal for others, the age-predicted HRmax estimates are relatively useless for clinical purposes. Estimates of HRmax should be only one of several indicators of maximal effort.
2. In a comprehensive review of more than 23,000 subjects ranging in age from 5 to 81 years,[7] a stepwise multiple regression showed that age alone accounted for 75% of the variability; other factors added only about 5% and included mode of exercise, level of fitness, and continent of origin. The 95% confidence interval, even when these factors were controlled, was 45 beats per minute. Heart rates at maximal exercise were lower on bicycle ergometry than on treadmill and lower still with swimming. Trained individuals had significantly lower maximal heart rates for their ages.
3. An important factor determining maximal exercise heart rate is motivation to exert oneself maximally.

Specific Heart Rate Responses

1. **Normal:** The normal rise should be progressive in proportion to the relative intensity of the workload. If the workload stays stable, heart rate will continue to rise slowly, probably due to a loss of intravascular volume.
2. **Blunted:** A lowered maximal heart rate is usually due to a beta blocker with a value of 110 to 120 if the medication is being taken regularly. Although calcium antagonists and digoxin decrease heart rate in patients with atrial fibrillation, they have little effect on exercise heart rate in patients in normal sinus rhythm.
3. **Deconditioned:** There is a fast initial rise in heart rate in response to relatively low workloads and an elevated maximal value. This same response occurs in patients experiencing atrial fibrillation who are not receiving rate-controlling medications.
4. **Disease states:** In addition to the associated deconditioning, patients with chronic illnesses, including anemia, will have excessive heart rate responses due to inadequate oxygen delivery or decreased cardiac output.

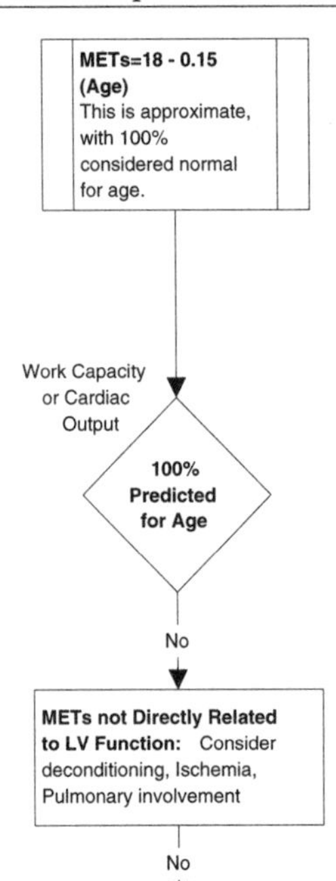

EXERCISE CAPACITY OR FUNCTIONAL CAPACITY

1. Maximal ventilatory oxygen uptake (Vo_2 max) is the greatest amount of oxygen that a person can extract from inspired air while performing dynamic exercise involving a large part of the total body muscle mass.
2. Because maximal ventilatory oxygen uptake is equal to the product of cardiac output and arterial venous oxygen (a-VO_2) difference, it is an indirect measure of the functional limits of the cardiovascualr system.
3. Maximal a-VO_2 difference is physiologically limited to roughly 15 to 17 vol% (i.e., a constant), making maximal oxygen uptake an indirect estimate of maximal cardiac output.

Factors Affecting Maximal Exercise Capacity

1. Maximal oxygen uptake depends on many factors, including natural physical endowment, activity status, age, and gender, but it is the best index of exercise capacity and maximal cardiovascular function.
2. Aerobic training can increase maximal oxygen uptake by up to 25%, and bed rest can do the converse. This increase is dependent on the initial level of fitness and

age, as well as on the intensity, frequency, and length of training sessions.

Exercise Capacity and Cardiac Function

1. Correlations between exercise capacity and various indices of ventricular function have been very poor, ranging from 0.10 to 0.24.[8]
2. Increasing heart rate and cardiac index appear to be the most important determinants of exercise capacity.
3. Good ventricular function does not guarantee normal exercise capacity, and the reverse is also true. Thus, even in patients free of angina, exercise limitations or expectations should not be determined by ventricular function but rather by a particular patient's symptomatic response to exercise.
4. Abnormal ventricular function does not mean that exercise capacity is abnormal; an exercise test must be performed to determine exercise capacity.

Specific Key Values for METS

1. Ventilatory oxygen consumption is expressed in multiples of basal resting requirements (METS). The MET is a unit of basal oxygen consumption equal to approximately 3.5 ml O_2/kg/min. This value is the average amount of oxygen from inspired air required to maintain life in the resting state.[9]
2. Key MET values are as follows:
   a. 5 METS or less is associated with a poor prognosis in patients younger than 65.
   b. 5 METS is the usual exercise limit in the immediate postmyocardial infarction period.
   c. 10 METS is considered an acceptable level of fitness; when found in an angina patient, there is no improvement in survival with coronary artery bypass surgery versus medical management.
   d. 13 METS indicates a good prognosis in spite of any abnormal exercise test responses.
   e. 22 METS can be achieved by well-trained aerobic athletes.

Use of Nomograms for Exercise Capacity

1. Since $\dot{V}O_2$ is dependent on age, gender, activity status, and disease states, tables are needed that consider these factors to categorize a certain MET value accurately as either normal or abnormal.

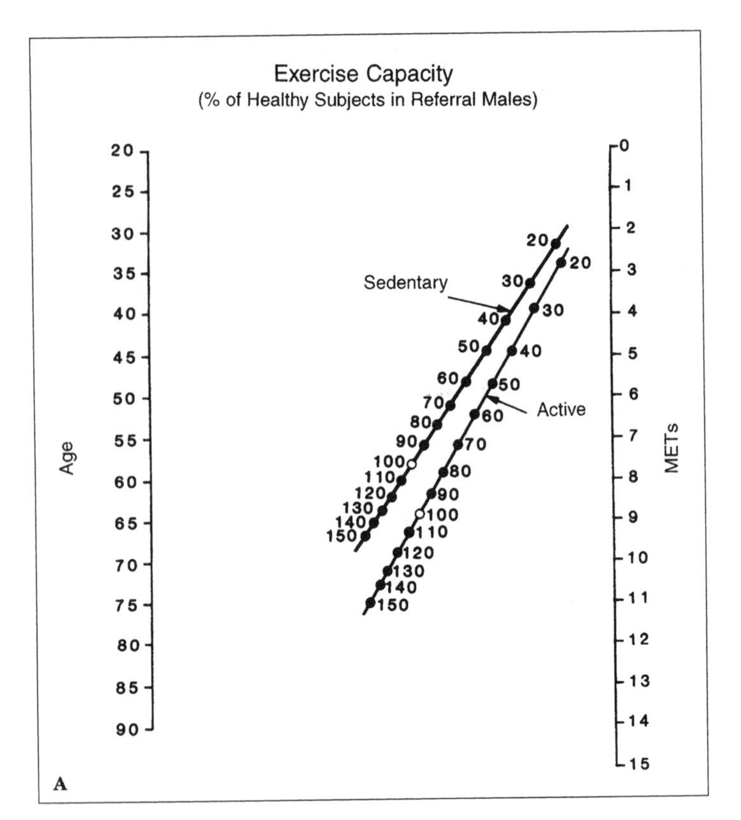

Fig. 14-2A and B. Aerobic nomograms considering exercise status for all referrals and normal subjects. One hundred percent is normal as expected for age.

2. Nomograms replace these tables by conveniently translating a MET level into a percentage of normal exercise capacity for males based on age and activity status (Fig. 14-2).[10]
3. Activity status is classified by asking, "Do you perform 20 minutes or more of brisk walking three times a week or regularly participate in an aerobic sport?"[11]
4. Separate nomograms were developed from healthy males who volunteered for maximal exercise testing with ventilatory gas exchange analysis. These subjects differed from the "normal" patients in that they were not referred for any clinical reason and were a healthy, younger, free-living population. They were also classified into sedentary and active groups.
5. The predicted METS for age were calculated by the

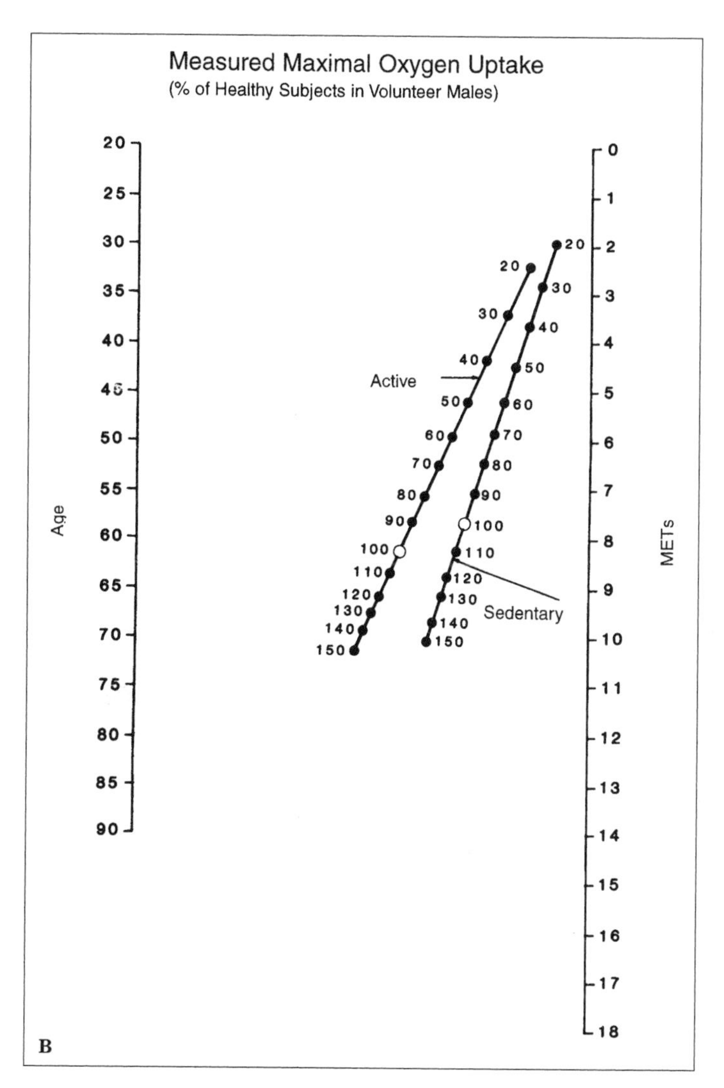

Fig. 14-2, *continued*

formulas obtained from the regression analysis using age as the independent variable. This was done for the entire group as well as for the Sedentary and Active groups separately. A percentage of exercise capacity was obtained from the following equation:

$$\text{exercise capacity} = \frac{\text{observed METS level}}{\text{predicted METS}} \times 100$$

6. Exercise capacity represents the actual percentage capacity for a given age based on METS performed, with 100% being the average for that age group.
7. Among patients tested for clinical reasons ("referrals"), regression analyses of METS against age for the entire group and for each of the two subgroups yielded the following equations:

All "referrals":	predicted METS = 18.0 − 0.15 (age)
Active:	predicted METS = 18.7 − 0.15 (age)
Sedentary:	predicted METS = 16.6 − 0.16 (age)

Regression analysis of METS against age for the healthy subjects and for active and sedentary subgroups yielded the following equations:

All (healthy subjects):	predicted METS = 14.7 − 0.11 (age)
Active:	predicted METS = 16.4 − 0.13 (age)
Sedentary:	predicted METS = 11.9 − 0.07 (age)

8. MET levels can be used for exercise prescription and for estimating levels of disability by using tables listing the MET demands for most common activities (Table 14-1).
9. The other major population studies yielded the following equation[12]:

predicted METS = 16.2 − 0.11 (age)

10. These nomograms are simple to use, requiring only values for age and observed MET levels to draw a line between them and obtain the percentage for normal exercise capacity.
11. For instance, if a patient completed 6 minutes of a Bruce protocol (Stage 2), he will have achieved an exercise capacity of 7 METS. If he is aged 55 years, this will calculate to an exercise capacity of 78% using the nomogram. Similarly, if the same patient completed 8 minutes of a Balke protocol, he will also have achieved 7 METS and have an exercise capacity of 78%.
12. Values below 100% indicate exercise impairment relative to one's age group, whereas values above 100% indicate supernormal performance.
13. Equations based on time in a protocol or other parameters can be used as follows.

Errata — *Handbook of Exercise Testing*

Fig. 5-1. The normal ECG response to treadmill exercise is illustrated. Note that there can be considerable normal ST junctional (junction of the QRS and ST wave forms) depression. (HR 120, average ECG at heart rate of 120 bpm.) These are averaged waveforms from the exercise tests of 50 normal subjects.

Fig. 5-5. This illustrates the points from which ST elevation or depression is measured if the standing ECG exhibits ST elevation (early repolarization as in A and B) or if the standing ECG exhibits ST segment depression (as in C and D). ***Note:*** **The ST depression is measured from the isoelectric line (not from the standing preexercise baseline) when ST elevation is present at rest (as in A, which occurs most commonly).**

Fig. 5-6. ST segment deviation assessment. Elevation over Q waves is diagnostic of myocardial infarction.

Table 14-1. METS Demands for Most Common Activities

Activity	*METS*	*Activity*	*METS*
Mild		***Vigorous***	
Baking	2.0	Badminton	5.5
Billiards	2.4	Chopping wood	4.9
Bookbinding	2.2	Climbing hills	7.0
Canoeing (leisurely)	2.5	Cycling (moderate)	5.7
Conducting an orchestra	2.2	Dancing	6.0
Dancing, ballroom (slow)	2.9	Field hockey	7.7
Golf (with cart)	2.5	Ice skating	5.5
Horseback riding (walking)	2.3	Jogging (10-minute mile)	10
Playing a musical instrument	2.0	Karate or judo	6.5
Volleyball (noncompetitive)	2.9	Roller skating	6.5
Walking (2 mph)	2.5	Rope skipping	12
Writing	1.7	Skiing (water or downhill)	6.8
		Squash	12
Moderate		Surfing	6.0
Calisthenics (no weights)	4.0	Swimming (fast)	7.0
Croquet	3.0	Tennis (doubles)	6.0
Cycling (leisurely)	3.5		
Gardening (no lifting)	4.4		
Golf (without cart)	4.9		
Mowing lawn (power mower)	3.0		
Playing drums	3.8		
Sailing	3.0		
Swimming (slowly)	4.5		
Walking (3 mph)	3.3		
Walking (4 mph)	4.5		

From American Heart Association. *Exercise standards.* Dallas: The Association, 1990.

For time in the Bruce protocol:

$$\text{METS} = 1.11 + 0.016\ (\text{duration in seconds})$$

For treadmill speed and grade:

$$\text{METS} = (\text{mph} \times 26.8) \times [0.1 + (\text{Grade} \times 0.018) + 3.5]/3.5$$

Ergometer workload:

$$\text{METS} = [(2 \times \text{kpm/min} + 300)/\text{body weight in kilograms}]/3.5$$

14. The total population nomograms are appropriate if activity status is unknown. The “referral” nomograms may be used for patients referred for testing for clinical reasons, and the nomograms of healthy subjects may be more appropriate for individuals tested for screening or preexercise program evaluations.

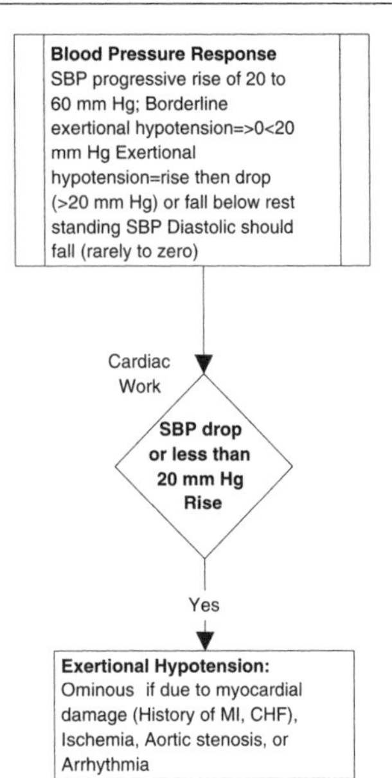

BLOOD PRESSURE RESPONSE

Normal Response

1. Systolic blood pressure should rise with increasing treadmill workload from 40 to 60 mm Hg. Maximal SBP should not be greater than 250 mm Hg.
2. Diastolic blood pressure usually remains unchanged and should not exceed 115 mm Hg, but the fifth Korotkoff sound can sometimes be heard all the way to zero in healthy young subjects. Although a rising diastolic blood pressure can be associated with coronary heart disease, it is more likely a marker for labile hypertension, which causes coronary disease.
3. The highest SBP should be achieved at maximal workload.
4. When exercise is stopped, approximately 10% of the individuals tested will abruptly drop their SBP because of peripheral pooling. To avoid fainting, patients should quickly be allowed to lie down.
5. The SBP usually normalizes on patients resuming the supine position during recovery but may remain below normal for several hours after the test.
6. The automated methods of measuring SBP have not been proven to be accurate. Although the available devices may correlate with manual methods, they have

not yet been adequately validated, particularly for the detection of exertional hypotension.

Exertional Hypotension

1. Exercise-induced hypotension (EIH) is defined as a failure of SBP to rise, a drop below standing rest prior to testing, or a drop of 20 mm Hg after a rise.
2. Exercise-induced hypotension has been demonstrated in most studies to predict either a poor prognosis or a high probability of severe angiographic coronary artery disease.
3. An abnormal SBP response has been found to indicate an increased risk of cardiac events.
4. Exercise-induced hypotension has been associated with cardiac complications during exercise testing and appears to be corrected by coronary artery bypass surgery.[13]
5. Even when tested to exhaustion, most healthy individuals do not exhibit any reduction in SBP. Exercise-induced hypotension occurs more frequently in healthy females than in males. Normally, after exercise, there is a drop in both systolic and diastolic pressure.
6. Exercise-induced hypotension can occur in patients with coronary artery disease, valvular heart disease, cardiomyopathies, and arrhythmias. Occasionally, patients without clinically significant heart disease will exhibit EIH during exercise due to antihypertensive therapy, including beta blockers, prolonged strenuous exercise, and vasovagal responses.
7. Exercise-induced hypotension can be due to chronic ventricular dysfunction, exercise-induced ischemia causing left ventricular dysfunction, or papillary muscle dysfunction and mitral regurgitation.[14]

DOUBLE PRODUCT

1. It has been shown that myocardial oxygen uptake is best estimated by the product of heart rate and SBP (double product).
2. Exercise-induced angina and ST depression usually occur at the same double product in an individual.
3. When this is not the case, the influence of other factors should be suspected such as a recent meal, abnormal ambient temperature, or coronary artery spasm.
4. This product is also an estimate of the maximal workload that the left ventricle can perform.

5. An adequate double product is a value greater than 25,000.

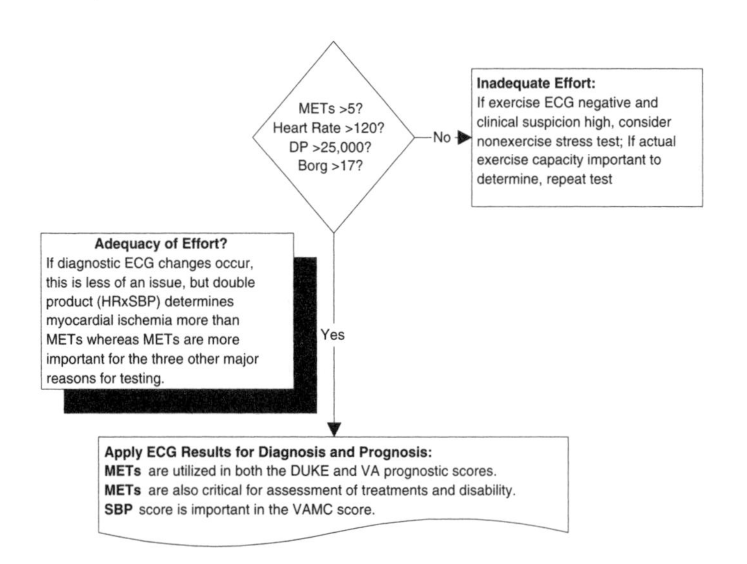

KEY POINTS IN INTERPRETATION OF HEMODYNAMIC RESPONSES

1. Because it can objectively demonstrate exercise capacity, exercise testing is used for disability evaluation in preference to relying on functional classifications. No questionnaire or submaximal test or nonexercise stress test can give the same results as a symptom-limited exercise test.
2. Age-predicted maximal heart rate targets are relatively useless for clinical purposes, and it is surprising how much steeper the age-related decline in maximal heart rate is in referred populations as compared with age-matched healthy subjects or volunteers. A consistent finding in population studies has been a relatively poor relationship between maximal heart rate and age. Correlation coefficients of −0.4 are usually found with a standard error of the estimate of 10 to 25 bpm.
3. Exertional hypotension, best defined as a drop in SBP below standing rest or a drop of 20 mm Hg after a rise, is predictive of severe angiographic coronary artery disease and a poor prognosis. A failure of SBP to rise is particularly worrisome after a myocardial infarction.
4. Until automated devices are adequately validated, we

strongly recommend that blood pressure be taken manually with a cuff and stethoscope.

5. The nomogram greatly facilitates the description of exercise capacity relative to age and enables comparison among patients. Reporting exercise capacity as a percentage, with 100% as normal for age, is highly recommended.

REFERENCES

1. Myers J, Froelicher VF. Hemodynamic determinants of exercise capacity in chronic heart failure. *Am Intern Med* 115:377–386, 1991.
2. McKirnan MD, Sullivan M, Jensen D, Froelicher VF. Treadmill performance and cardiac function in selected patients with coronary heart disease. *J Am Coll Cardiol* 3:253–261, 1984.
3. Hammond HK, Kelley TL, Froelicher VF. Noninvasive testing in the evaluation of myocardial ischemia: Agreement among tests. *J Am Coll Cardiol* 5:59–69, 1985.
4. Hammond K, Froelicher VF. Normal and abnormal heart rate responses to exercise. *Prog Cardiol Dis* 27:271–296, 1985.
5. Convertino V, Hung J, Goldwater D, Watson A, Dimars T. Cardiovascular responses to exercise in middle-aged man after 10 days of bedrest. *Circulation* 65:134–140, 1982.
6. Hammond HK, Kelley TL, Froelicher V. Radionuclide imaging correlatives of heart rate impairment during maximal exercise testing. *J Am Coll Cardiol* 2(5): 826–833, 1983.
7. Londeree BR, Moeschberger ML. Influence of age and other factors on maximal heart rate. *J Cardiac Rehab* 4:44–49, 1984.
8. McKirnan D, Sullivan M, Jensen D, Froelicher VF. Treadmill performance and cardial function in selected patients with coronary heart disease. *J Am Coll Cardiol* 3:253–261, 1984.
9. Froelicher VF, Thompson AJ, Noquero I, Davis G, Stewart A, Triebwasser J. Prediction of maximal oxygen consumption: Comparison of the Bruce and Balke treadmill protocols. *Chest* 68:331–336, 1975.
10. Morris C, Myers J, Kawaguchi T, Heshima K, Hideg A, Froelicher VF. Nomogram for exercise capacity using METs and age. *J Am Coll Cardiol* 22:175–182, 1993.

11. Morris CK, Ueshima K, Kawaguchi T, Hideg A, Froelicher VF. The prognostic value of exercise capacity: A review of the literature. *Am Heart J* 122:1423–1430, 1991.
12. Dehn MM, Bruce RA. Longitudinal variations in maximal oxygen intake with age and activity. *J Appl Physiol* 33:805–807, 1972.
13. Morris SN, Phillips JF, Jordan JW, McHenry PL. Incidence of significance of decreases in systolic blood pressure during graded treadmill exercise testing. *Am J Cardiol* 41:221–226, 1978.
14. Irving JB, Bruce RA. Exertional hypotension and postexertional ventricular fibrillation in stress testing. *Am J Cardiol* 39(6):849–851, 1977.

ECG Responses

THE NORMAL ELECTROCARDIOGRAPHIC RESPONSE TO EXERCISE

The exercise ECG response will be presented in the sequence of the ECG waveforms.[1]

P Wave

1. The P wave usually has only minor changes during exercise, and the appearance of P pulmonale or P mitrale is rare and of questionable significance.
2. The effect of atrial repolarization on the ST-segments in the lateral leads (V_4, V_5, V_6) is minimal, but it affects inferior leads (II, AVF, III) and is particularly noticeable when the PR interval is short. This can cause a false-positive test.[2,3]

Q-Wave, R-Wave, and S-Wave Amplitudes

1. As the R wave decreases in amplitude, the S wave increases in depth.
2. QRS duration tends to decrease with exercise and increasing heart rate in healthy subjects and increase in patients with either angina or left ventricular dysfunction.[4,5] However, there is too much overlap in QRS duration responses to permit discrimination between them.

R-Wave Changes

1. R-wave amplitude typically increases from rest to submaximal exercise, perhaps to a heart rate of 130 bpm, and then decreases to a minimum at maximal exercise.
2. If a patient is limited by objective or subjective symptoms or signs, the R-wave amplitude will increase from rest to such an endpoint. Such patients may be demonstrating a normal R-wave response but be classified as "abnormal" because of a submaximal effort.
3. Exercise-induced changes in R-wave amplitude have no independent predictive power but are associated with coronary artery disease because such patients are often submaximally tested and an R-wave decrease normally occurs at maximal exercise.
4. A multitude of factors affect the R-wave amplitude re-

sponse to exercise, and the response does not have diagnostic significance.[6]

ST Slope, J-Junction Depression, and T-Wave Amplitude

1. There is depression of the J junction and tall, peaked T waves at maximal exercise and at 1 minute recovery in healthy subjects. Along with the J-junction depression, there can be marked ST upsloping.
2. Junctional depression is the result of competition between normal repolarization and delayed terminal depolarization forces.
3. A gradual decrease in T-wave amplitude is normally observed in all leads during early exercise.

U-Wave Changes

Ischemia is rarely associated with inversion of U waves. When this occurs, it usually is in the anterior precordial leads.[7]

ABNORMAL ST-SEGMENT CHANGES

General Methods

1. Always consider the resting ECG configuration and the ST level during standing rest before the test.
2. V_5 remains the single most important lead for clinically significant ST changes during exercise, except when the ECG is distorted by diagnostic Q waves.
3. When the resting ECG is normal, ST depression isolated to the inferior leads (II, III, AVF) is usually indicative of a false positive.
4. On the surface electrocardiogram, exercise-induced myocardial ischemia can result in one of three ST-segment manifestations:
   a. Elevation
   b. Normalization
   c. Depression

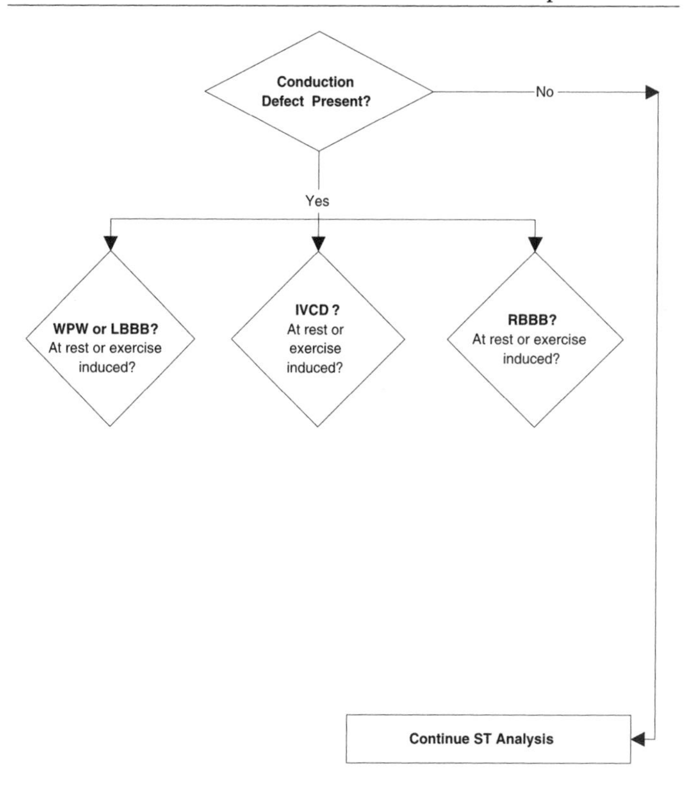

Conduction Defects

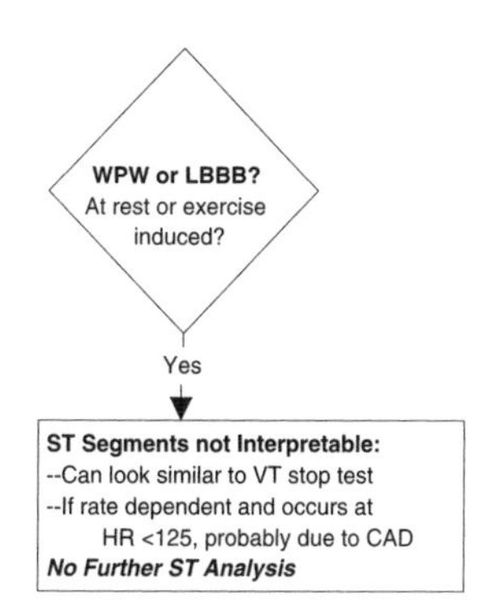

Left Bundle Branch Block

1. The ST-segment response to exercise testing cannot be used to make diagnostic decisions on patients with left bundle branch block (LBBB).[8] Even a centimeter of depression can occur in healthy individuals.

2. When exercise-induced heart rate-dependent LBBB[9] occurs at a heart rate of 125 bpm or less, coronary artery disease should be suspected.

Wolfe-Parkinson-White Syndrome

1. This rare pattern on the ECG negates the ST response during exercise of any association with ischemia.
2. It can be affected by exercise in several ways: it can be induced by exercise and appear to be ventricular tachycardia or it can disappear during exercise and be replaced with a normal pattern.

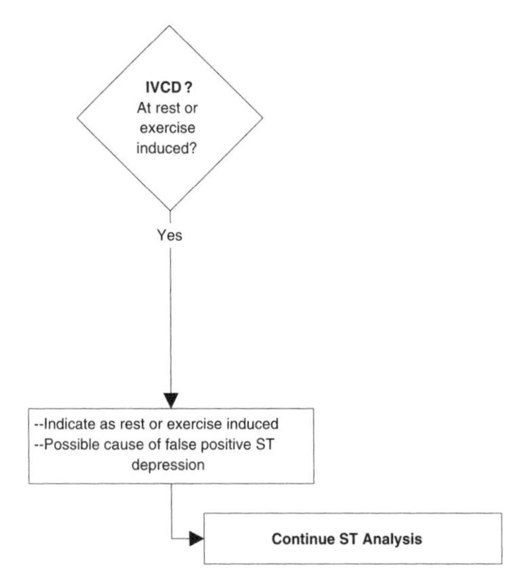

Intraventricular Conduction Defect

1. Prolongation of the QRS complex to 120 msec without the appearance of either type of bundle branch block can occur on the resting ECG or be induced by tachycardia.
2. Drugs such as quinidine can cause this as well.
3. IVCD can be associated with a false-positive response, particularly when accompanied by ST depression at rest.

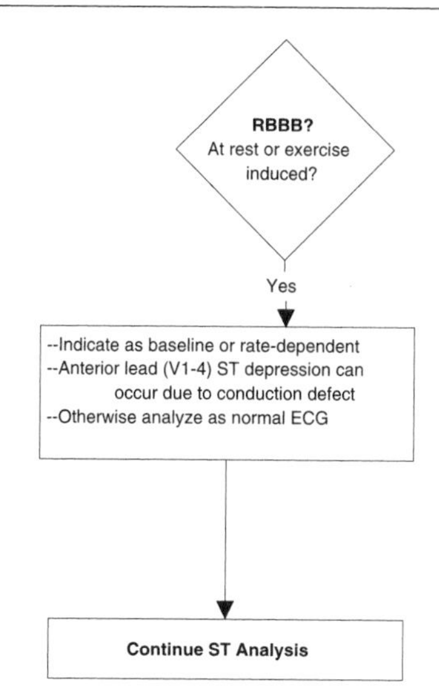

Right Bundle Branch Block

1. In healthy men with acquired right bundle branch block (RBBB),[10] there is no exercise-induced ST-segment depression in the inferior and lateral leads, although depression in the anterior precordial leads is frequently noted.
2. This is most apparent in the right precordial leads with an rSR′ or a notched R wave; these leads often show a down-sloping ST segment at rest, and such a finding is thus not indicative of myocardial ischemia.
3. ST depression occurring in V_5 or V_6 is associated with ischemia as in a normal ECG.

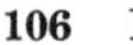

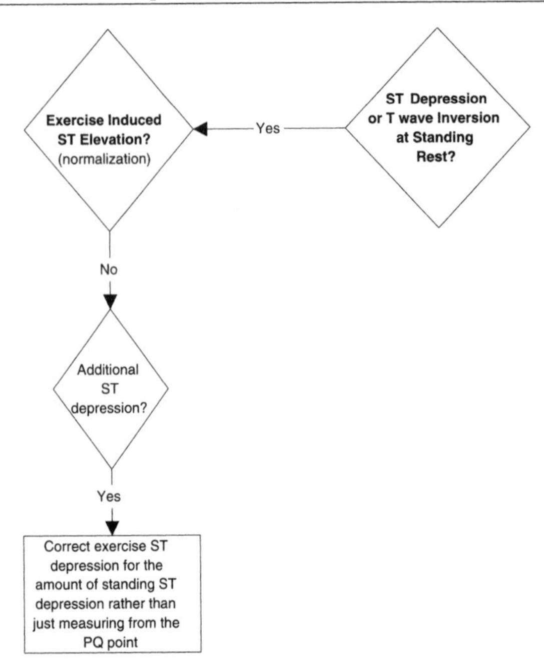

Baseline ST-Segment Depression

1. Isolated ST depression on the resting ECG and left ventricular hypertrophy with strain are associated with an increased risk of cardiac events and angiographically significant coronary disease.
2. It was once thought that these abnormalities negate the value of the standard exercise test because of a decrease in specificity. However, the standard test remains the best first test for patients with these abnormalities because sensitivity is unaffected.
3. Exercise-induced ST depression is measured from the level of ST depression noted at standing rest, and a 2-mm additional depression criterion maintains good diagnostic characteristics.

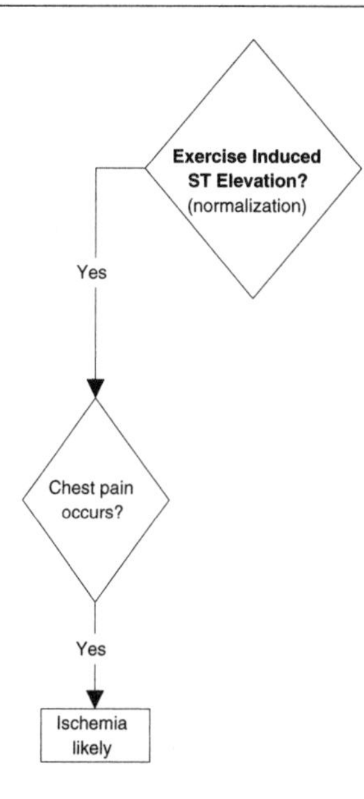

ST-SEGMENT NORMALIZATION

1. Another manifestation of ischemia can be either no change or normalization of the ST segment due to cancellation effects. A patient can have his or her "best"-looking ECG during ischemia!
2. Electrocardiographic abnormalities at rest, including T-wave inversion and ST-segment depression, can return to normal during attacks of angina and during exercise in some patients with ischemic heart disease.
3. This cancellation effect is a rare occurrence, but it should be considered. This normalization of ST-segment depression is probably ST-segment elevation associated with transmural ischemia.[11]
4. Pseudo-normalization is not meaningful without pain, and, in fact, ischemia can only be identified when chest pain consistent with angina occurs as well.

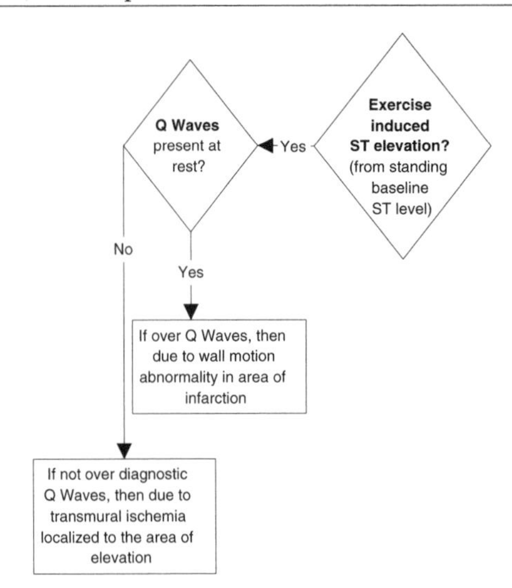

ST-SEGMENT ELEVATION

Prevalence of Exercise-induced ST Elevation

The most common electrocardiogram abnormality seen in the exercise laboratory is ST-segment depression. ST elevation is relatively common after a Q-wave infarction, but ST elevation without Q waves occurs in only one out of a thousand patients.[12-14]

Methods of Measuring ST Elevation

1. ST-segment elevation is always measured from the baseline ST level. It is important to differentiate elevation occurring over, or adjacent to, Q waves from elevation in non-Q-wave areas.
2. Left ventricular aneurysm after myocardial infarction is the most frequent cause of ST-segment elevation on the resting electrocardiogram and occurs over Q waves or in electrocardiographic leads adjacent to Q waves. ST elevation normally occurs over diagnostic Q waves and is very common after a recent myocardial infarction.
3. Early repolarization is a normal resting pattern of ST elevation that occurs in healthy subjects who do not have diagnostic Q waves. The ST level at rest with early repolarization normally sinks down to the isoelectric line with an increase in heart rate.
4. ST elevation on a normal ECG (other than in AVR or V_1) represents transmural ischemia, is very rare (0.1%

in a clinical laboratory), is very arrythmogenic, and localizes the ischemia. When it occurs in V_2 to V_4, the left anterior descending is involved, when in the lateral leads the left circumflex and diagonals are involved, and when in II, III, and AVF the right coronary artery is involved.

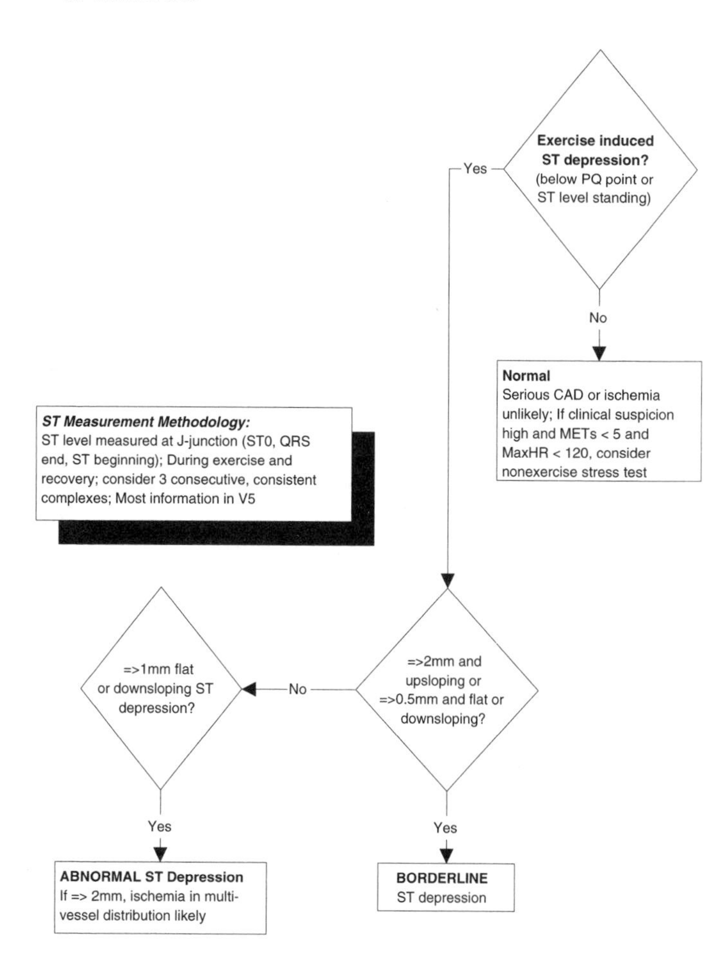

ST-SEGMENT DEPRESSION

1. The most common manifestation of exercise-induced myocardial ischemia is ST-segment depression.
2. The standard criterion for this type of abnormal response is horizontal or downward-sloping ST-segment depression of 0.1 mV or more for 60 msec.

3. ST-segment depression is measured from the isoelectric baseline. When ST-segment depression is present at rest, the amount of additional depression is measured.
4. It appears to be due to generalized subendocardial ischemia. A "steal" phenomenon is likely from ischemic areas because of the effect of extensive collateralization in the subendocardium.
5. ST depression does not localize the area of ischemia or indicate which coronary artery is occluded.
6. The normal ST-segment vector response to tachycardia and to exercise is a shift rightward and upward. The degree of this shift appears to have a fair amount of biological variation. Most healthy subjects will have early repolarization at rest, which will shift to the isoelectric PR-segment line in the inferior, lateral, and anterior leads with exercise. This shift can be further influenced by ischemia and myocardial scars. When the latter portions of the ST segment are affected, flattening or downward depression can be recorded.
7. The more leads with these apparent ischemic shifts, the more severe the disease.
8. The probability and severity of coronary artery disease are directly related to the amount of J-junction depression, the number of leads involved, and the duration of the depression in recovery. They are inversely related to the slope of the ST-segment and to the heart rate, systolic blood pressure (double product), and the METS at the time the depression appears during exercise.
9. Downward-sloping ST-segment depression is more serious than horizontal depression, and both are more serious than upward-sloping depression. However, patients with upward-sloping ST-segment depression, especially when the slope is less than 1 mV/sec, probably have an increased probability of coronary disease.
10. If a slowly ascending slope is used as a criterion for abnormal, the specificity of exercise testing will be decreased (more false-positive results), although the test becomes more sensitive.
11. One electrode can show upward-sloping ST depression, whereas an adjacent electrode shows horizontal or downward-sloping depression.
12. If an apparently borderline ST segment, with an inad-

equate slope, is recorded in a single precordial lead in a patient highly suspected of having coronary artery disease, multiple precordial leads should be scanned before the exercise test is called normal.

13. An upward-sloping depressed ST segment may be the precursor to abnormal ST-segment depression in the recovery period or at higher heart rates during greater workloads.
14. The probability of ischemia and the likelihood of coronary artery disease severity are directly related to the amount of abnormal ST depression and inversely related to the slope (i.e., downward-sloping ST depression is the most serious and upward-sloping is the least serious).

ST Depression in Recovery

1. Abnormal ST depression occurring only in recovery provides clinically useful information and is not more likely to represent a false-positive response.
2. When considered together with changes in exercise, changes in recovery increase the sensitivity of the exercise test without a decline in predictive value.
3. A cool-down walk should be avoided after exercise testing, and the patient placed supine as soon as possible. Exercise test scores and nuclear testing should consider recovery ST measurements for evaluation.
4. Avoidance of a cool-down walk has not resulted in an increased complication rate.

ST Shift Location and Ischemia

1. ST depression is due to global subendocardial ischemia and does not localize on the surface ECG because the ST vector is directed up the long axis of the ventricle.
2. The leads exhibiting depression do not indicate which coronary artery is occluded. In fact, depression isolated to the inferior leads is usually a false-positive response.
3. V_5 is the lead predominately exhibiting significant ST depression. Depression isolated to other leads is usually due to Q-wave distortion of the resting ECG.
4. ST depression in the inferior leads (II, AVF) is most often due to the atrial repolarization wave, which begins in the PR segment and can extend to the beginning of the ST segment. When ST depression is isolated to these leads and there are no diagnostic Q waves, it is usually a false positive.

Exercise-induced ST-Segment Depression Not Due to Coronary Artery Disease

1. In a population with a high prevalence of heart disease other than coronary artery disease, an abnormal exercise test would be as diagnostic for that disease as it would be for coronary artery disease in populations with a high prevalence of coronary artery disease.
2. Digitalis, and possibly some psychotropic drugs, can cause exercise-induced repolarization abnormalities in healthy subjects.
3. Patients who have had abnormal responses, and who have anemia or electrolyte abnormalities or are on medications, should be retested when these conditions are altered.
4. Meals and even glucose ingestion can alter the ST segment and T wave in the resting ECG and can potentially cause a false-positive response. To avoid this problem, all electrocardiographic studies should be performed after at least a 4-hour fast. Exercise capacity is decreased after eating because cardiac output is diverted to the GI tract. If cardiac output is not adequate, angina occurs at a lower exercise stress than usual. In addition, CPR is safer on an empty stomach.

Table 15-1 lists some of the conditions that may result in false-positive responses.

Factors Related to False-positive ST Responses

GENDER

1. The specificity of the ST response is lower for women

Table 15-1. Conditions Associated with False-Positive ST-Exercise Responses

Valvular and congenital heart disease
Cardiomyopathies
Pericardial disease
Digoxin
Female gender
Electrolyte abnormalities
Not fasting prior to testing
Anemia
Inadequate ECG recorder
Bundle branch block (see text)
Improper ECG reading or incorrect criteria
Left ventricular hypertrophy or Wolff-Parkinson-White Syndrome
Preexcitation with short PR interval (ST depression due to atrial depolarization)
Mitral valve prolapse
Orthostatic abnormality
Hyperventilation (see text)
Improper leads

(but not for the sensitivity), and this is not explained entirely by hormones. Estrogen given to men does not increase the rate of false-positive responses.

2. The lower specificity of exercise-induced ST-segment depression in women could be due to hemodynamic or hemoglobin concentration differences.[15]

DIGOXIN

1. Administration of digoxin induces significant ST-T depression at rest and during exercise even at small doses.[16]
2. The most pronounced ST depression occurs at a heart rate of 110 to 130 bpm. At higher heart rates, the ST depression is less pronounced.
3. During the first minutes after exercise, no significant digitalis-induced ST-T depression is seen.
4. This pattern of ST depression associated with digoxin is not usually seen in myocardial ischemia.
5. Up to 14 days after withdrawal of digoxin, digitalis-induced ST-T changes are still apparent.

LEFT VENTRICULAR HYPERTROPHY WITH STRAIN. Individuals with left ventricular hypertrophy and strain pattern on their resting ECG are at high risk for coronary artery disease, but the ST response is less specific because of the association with diseases other than coronary disease.

WOLFF-PARKINSON-WHITE. Healthy individuals with the Wolff-Parkinson-White syndrome can have exercise-induced ST-segment depression. Some individuals with the preexcitation, a short PR interval, and a normal QRS complex may have a false-positive exercise test.

MITRAL VALVE PROLAPSE. Patients with prolapsing mitral valve syndrome can have abnormal exercise tests but normal coronary angiograms. In individuals with this syndrome, false-positive responses are apparently more common, occurring in approximately 25%.

ORTHOSTATIC ST CHANGES. Some individuals with ST depression induced by standing can have abnormal exercise-induced ST-segment changes without coronary artery disease. This is also the case for those with hyperventilation repolarization changes. Such changes are unusual and have rarely been responsible for false-positive tests. Orthostatic and hyperventilation ST changes have been associated with the mitral valve prolapse syndrome.

EXERCISE-INDUCED VENTRICULAR ARRHYTHMIAS

1. Ventricular arrhythmias in general do not have the same significance in the exercise lab as they do in the

cardiac care unit. They increase in frequency and prevalence with age. In the exercise laboratory, they are usually ominous only when they occur in patients with a history of sudden death, cardiomyopathy, valvular heart disease, or severe ischemia (particularly ST elevation with a normal resting ECG).
2. As with resting ventricular arrhythmias, the significance of exercise-induced ventricular arrhythmias is related to the disease processes with which they are associated (history of syncope, sudden death, or physical examination with cardiomegaly, murmurs; ECG showing prolonged QT, preexcitation, Q-waves). If there are no signs or symptoms of associated disease, exercise-induced ventricular arrhythmias can usually be ignored (Don't behave like you are in a CCU!).
3. Exercise-induced ventricular arrhythmias increase with age but do not have an independent association with death in most patients with coronary disease; that is, other variables are better predictors.
4. There is a small percentage of patients in whom exercise-induced ventricular arrhythmias are independently predictive of death.

Ventricular Tachycardia during Exercise Testing

1. Nonsustained ventricular tachycardia is uncommon during routine clinical treadmill testing (prevalence less than 2%), is well tolerated, and has a prognosis determined by the accompanying ischemia and left ventricular damage.
2. It is limited to short, asymptomatic runs of 3 to 6 beats, usually near peak exercise, and does not predict increased cardiovascular morbidity or mortality.[17-19]

REFERENCES

1. Wolthuis RA, Froelicher VF, Hopkirk A, Longo M, Lemeister M. Normal electrocardiographic waveform characteristics during treadmill exercise testing. *Circulation* 60:1028–1035, 1979.
2. Riff DP, Carleton RA. Effect of exercise on the atrial recovery wave. *Am Heart J* 82:759–763, 1971.
3. Sapin PM, Koch G, Blauwet MB, McCarthy JJ, Hinds SW, Gettes LS. Identification of false positive exercise tests with use of electrocardiographic criteria: A possible role for atrial repolarization waves. *J Am Coll Cardiol* 18:127–135, 1991.
4. Ahnve S, Sullivan M, Myers J, Froelicher V. Com-

puter analysis of exercise-induced changes in QRS duration in patients with angina pectoris and in normal subjects. *Am Heart J* 111(5):903–908, 1986.
5. Goldberger AL, Bhargava V. Effect of exercise on QRS duration in healthy men: A computer ECG analysis. *J Appl Physiol* 54(4):1083–1088, 1983.
6. Myers J, Ahnve S, Froelicher V, Sullivan M. Spatial R wave amplitude during exercise: Relation with left ventricular ischemia and function. *J Am Coll Cardiol* 6:603–608, 1985.
7. Gerson MC, Morris SN, McHenry PL. Relation of exercise induced physiologic ST segment depression to R wave amplitude in normal subjects. *Am J Cardiol* 46:778–782, 1980.
8. Whinnery JE, Froelicher VF, Stuart AJ. The electrocardiographic response to maximal treadmill exercise in asymptomatic men with left bundle branch block. *Am Heart J* 94:316, 1977.
9. Vasey CG, O'Donnell J, Morris SN, McHenry P. Exercise-induced left bundle branch block and its relation to coronary artery disease. *Am J Cardiol* 56:892–895, 1985.
10. Whinnery JE, Froelicher VF, Stuart AJ. The electrocardiographic response to maximal treadmill exercise in asymptomatic men with right branch bundle block. *Chest* 71:335, 1977.
11. Lavie CJ, Oh JK, Mankin HT, Clements IP, Giuliani ER, Gibbons RJ. Significance of T-wave pseudonormalization during exercise: A radionuclide angiographic study. *Chest* 94:512–516, 1988.
12. Fortuin NJ, Friesinger GC. Exercise-induced ST segment elevation: Clinical, electrocardiographic and arteriographic studies in twelve patients. *Am J Med* 49:459, 1970.
13. Hegge FN, Tuna N, Burchell HB. Coronary arteriographic findings in patients with axis shifts or ST segment elevations on exercise testing. *Am Heart J* 86:603, 1973.
14. Chahine RA, Raizner AE, Ishimori T. The clinical significance of exercise-induced ST-segment elevation. *Circulation* 54:209, 1976.
15. Robert AR, Melin JA, Detry JM. Logistic discriminant analysis improves diagnostic accuracy of exercise testing for coronary artery disease in women. *Circulation* 83(4):1202–1209, 1991.
16. Sundqvist K, Atterhog JH, Jogestrand T. Effect of di-

goxin on the electrocardiogram at rest and during exercise in healthy subjects. *Am J Cardiol* 57:661–665, 1986.

17. Yang JC, Wesley RC, Froelicher VF. Ventricular tachycardia during routine treadmill testing: Risk and prognosis. *Arch Intern Med* 151:349–353, 1991.
18. Detry JR, Mengeot P, Ronsseau MF, Cosyns J, Ponlot R, Biasseur LA. Maximal exercise testing in patients with spontaneous angina pectoris associated with transient ST segment elevation: Risks and electrocardiographic findings. *Br Heart J* 37:897–905, 1975.
19. Fleg JL, Lakatta EG. Prevalence and prognosis of exercise-induced nonsustained ventricular tachycardia in apparently healthy volunteers. *Am J Cardiol* 54: 762, 1984.

Key Points from Part III

Because it can objectively demonstrate exercise capacity, exercise testing is used for disability evaluation rather than relying on functional classifications. No questionnaire or submaximal test can give as accurate results as a symptom-limited exercise test.

Age-predicted maximal heart rate targets are relatively useless for clinical purposes, and it is surprising how much steeper the age-related decline in maximal heart rate is in referred populations compared with age-matched healthy subjects or volunteers. A consistent finding in population studies has been a relatively poor relationship of maximal heart rate to age. Correlation coefficients of −0.4 are usually found with a standard error of the estimate of 10 to 25 bpm.

Exertional hypotension, best defined as a drop in systolic blood pressure below standing rest or a drop of 20 mm Hg after a rise, is very predictive of severe angiographic coronary artery disease and a poor prognosis. A failure of systolic blood pressure to rise is particularly worrisome after a myocardial infarction.

Until automated devices are adequately validated, we strongly recommend that blood pressure be taken manually with a cuff and a stethoscope.

The nomogram greatly facilitates the description of exercise capacity relative to age and enables comparison between patients. Reporting exercise capacity as a percentage with 100% as normal for age is highly recommended.

ST-segment depression is a representation of global subendocardial ischemia, with a direction determined largely by the placement of the heart in the chest. ST-segment depression does not localize coronary artery lesions.

V5 is the lead that predominates in exhibition of significant ST depression. Depression isolated to other leads is usually due to Q-wave distortion of the resting ECG.

ST depression in the inferior leads (II, AVF) is most often due to the atrial repolarization wave, which begins in the PR segment and can extend to the beginning of the ST segment. When ST depression is isolated to these inferior leads and there are no diagnostic Q waves, it is usually a false positive.

When the resting ECG shows Q waves of an old myocardial infarction, ST elevation is due to wall motion abnormalities, whereas accompanying ST depression can be due to a second area of ischemia or reciprocal changes. When the resting ECG results are normal, ST elevation is due to severe ischemia (spasm or a critical lesion), although accompanying ST depression is reciprocal. Such ST elevation is uncommon, very arrhythmogenic, and localizes the involved coronary artery.

Exercise-induced R-wave and S-wave amplitude changes do not correlate with changes in left ventricular volume, ejection fraction, or ischemia. The consensus of many studies is that such changes do not have diagnostic value.

ST-segment depression limited to the recovery period does not generally represent a "false-positive" response. Inclusion of analysis during this time increases the diagnostic yield of the exercise test.

Nonsustained ventricular tachycardia is uncommon during routine clinical treadmill testing (prevalence less than 2%) and is well tolerated. Its prognosis is determined by the accompanying ischemia and left ventricular damage.

Exercise-induced ST elevation (not over diagnostic Q waves) and ST depression both represent ischemia, but they are quite distinctive: **elevation** is due to transmural ischemia, is arrhythmogenic, has a 0.1% prevalence, and localizes the artery where there is spasm or a tight lesion, whereas **depression** is due to subendocardial ischemia, is not arrhythmogenic, has a 5% to 50% prevalence, is rarely due to spasm, and does not localize.

Applications of Exercise Testing

Diagnostic Applications

The exercise test should be used for diagnosis if the diagnosis of coronary artery disease is uncertain. Did the patient have any of the following prior to the test?

Symptoms or signs of coronary artery disease
Exercise-induced symptoms including syncope, near syncope, or palpitations
Chest pain
Old or new ECG abnormalities
Cardiac risk factors/markers
Hospitalization or observation to rule out myocardial infarction (MI) or unstable angina

If **Yes,** the test should be performed for diagnosis.

IS THE EXERCISE TEST A VALID DIAGNOSTIC PROCEDURE?

Believability Criteria for Diagnostic Tests

Certain criteria must be applied to judge the credibility and applicability of the results of studies evaluating diagnostic tests.[1] If these have not been followed, the test should not be used for this purpose. Patient selection identifying these two groups can be problematic.

First, the evaluation must include clearly defined comparison groups, one free of the disease being studied and one with the disease.

Patient Selection

The studies should include consecutive patients or randomly selected patients in whom the diagnosis is in doubt. Any diagnostic test appears to function well if obviously healthy subjects are compared with those who obviously have the disease in question. In most cases, sophisticated testing is not needed to differentiate the healthy population from the diseased. The issue is to evaluate patients who are suspected but not known to have the disease of interest and to differentiate those who do from those who do not. If the patients enrolled in the study do not represent this "diagnostic dilemma" group, the test may perform well in the study, but may not perform well in clinical practice.

Definition of Normals

A problem with determining specificity is including enough normals and the problem of the definition of normals.[2] Should subjects be low-risk individuals or patients without significant angiographic disease?[3,4] If low-risk subjects are used, the problem of limited challenge must be confronted and maximal heart rate is higher relative to age than for a patient group. The heart rate difference makes heart rate appear to be a much more useful discriminator than it is in a clinical population.

Inclusion of Diseased Patients

Problems arise in including patients who most certainly have the disease (i.e., post-MI patients) in this diagnostic sample. They may be included in studies to predict disease severity but should not be included in studies attempting to distinguish those with disease from those without disease.

The **second** "believability" criterion requires an independent, "blind" comparison of the test with the performance of a "gold" standard. The "gold" standard really should measure a clinically important state. For example, cardiac catheterization is used as the gold standard for coronary artery disease rather than symptoms of chest pain alone or another noninvasive test.

1. The gold standard result should not be available to those interpreting the test.
2. Also, if the gold standard requires subjective interpretation (as would be the case even for coronary angiography), the interpreter should not know the test result. Blinding the interpreters of the test to the gold standard and vice versa minimizes the risk of bias.
3. **If these criteria are met,** the study can be used as a basis for utilization of the test in clinical practice. To apply the test properly to patients, the following must be considered: Most tests merely indicate an increase or decrease in the probability of disease being present or not. To apply imperfect tests appropriately, you must estimate the probability of disease before the test is done ("pretest probability"), and then revise this probability according to the test result.

Meta-analysis of Diagnostic Studies

1. The variability of the reported diagnostic accuracy of the exercise electrocardiogram has been studied by

applying meta-analysis confirming that exercise testing can be believed as a diagnostic procedure.[5]

2. One hundred forty-seven consecutively published reports, involving 24,074 patients who underwent both coronary angiography and exercise testing, revealed a wide variability in sensitivity and specificity (the mean sensitivity was 66% with a range of 23% to 100% and a standard deviation of 16%; the mean specificity was 84%, with a range of 17% to 100% and a standard deviation of 17%).

Sensitivity from Meta-analysis

The percentage of those with coronary disease who had an abnormal ST response was found to be significantly and independently related to four study characteristics:

1. Sensitivity decreased when equivocal tests were considered normal.
2. Comparison with a "better" test (i.e., thallium scintigraphy) lowered the sensitivity of the exercise ECG.
3. Exclusion of patients on digitalis was associated with improved sensitivity.
4. Publication year: An increase in sensitivity and decrease in specificity were noted over the years the exercise test has been used. This may be because as clinicians become more familiar with a test and increasingly trust its results, they allow its results to influence the decision to perform angiography.

Specificity from Meta-analysis

The percentage of those without coronary disease that had a normal ST response has been found to be significantly and independently related to four variables:

1. When upward-sloping ST depression was classified as abnormal, specificity was lowered.
2. The exclusion of patients with prior MI was associated with a decreased specificity.
3. The specificity increased when patients with left bundle branch block were excluded.
4. The use of preexercise hyperventilation was associated with a decreased specificity.

The wide variability in test performance makes it important that clinicians apply rigorous control of the methods they use for testing and analysis. Upward-sloping ST depression should be consid-

ered borderline or negative, and hyperventilation should not be performed prior to testing.

DIAGNOSTIC CHARACTERISTICS AND TEST PERFORMANCE

Sensitivity and Specificity

1. Sensitivity is the percentage of patients with a disease who will have abnormal test results.
2. Specificity is the percentage of patients free of disease who will have normal test results.
3. The method of calculating these terms is shown in Fig. 16-1.

Cut Point or Discriminate Value

1. A basic step in applying any testing procedure for the separation of normals from patients with disease is to determine a value measured by the test that best separates the two groups.
2. The problem with any diagnostic test is that there is a large overlap in measurement values of a test in the groups with and without disease. All of the tests used for the diagnosis of coronary artery disease have a considerable overlap in the range of measurements for the normal population and for those with heart disease.
3. Problems arise when a certain value is used to separate these two groups (i.e., 0.1 mV of ST-segment depression). If the value is set far to the right (i.e., 0.2

$$\text{Sensitivity} = \frac{TP}{TP + FN} \times 100$$

$$\text{Specificity} = \frac{TN}{FP + TN} \times 100$$

$$\text{Relative risk}^{*} = \frac{\dfrac{TP}{TP + FP}}{\dfrac{FN}{TN + FN}}$$

$$\text{Predictive value of abnormal test}^{\dagger} = \frac{TP}{TP + FP} \times 100$$

Fig. 16-1. Definitions and calculation of sensitivity, specificity, predictive value, and risk ratio of a test. FN, false negatives, or those with normal test results and with disease; FP, false positives, or those with abnormal test results and no disease; TN, true negatives, or those with normal test results and no disease; TP, True positives, or those with abnormal test results and disease.

***Relative risk, or risk ratio, is the relative rate of occurrence of a disease in the group with an abnormal test result compared with those with a normal test result.**

†Predictive value of an abnormal response is the percentage of individuals with an abnormal test result who have disease.

mV of ST-segment depression) to identify nearly all the normals as being free of disease, giving the test a high specificity, the result will be that a substantial number of those with the disease will be found to have normal test results. If a value is chosen far to the left (i.e., 0.5 mm ST-segment depression) that identifies nearly all those with disease as having abnormal test results, giving the test a high sensitivity, then many normals will be identified as having abnormal test results. If a value is chosen that equally mislabels the normals and those with disease, the test will have its highest predictive accuracy.

4. There may be reasons for wanting to adjust a test to have a relatively higher sensitivity or relatively higher specificity than possible when predictive accuracy is optimal.
5. Sensitivity and specificity are inversely related: When sensitivity is highest, specificity is lowest and vice versa. Any test has a range of inversely related sensitivities and specificities that can be chosen by choosing a different discriminate or diagnostic value. These can be plotted as range of characteristic (ROC) curves.

Range of Characteristic Curves

1. Plots of sensitivity versus specificity for a range of measurement cut points provides an efficient way to compare test performance.
2. They are particularly helpful when optimal cut points for discriminating those with disease from those without disease are not established. An optimal cut point can be chosen along the plotted line.
3. A straight diagonal line indicates that the measurement or test has no discriminating power for the disease being tested.
4. The greater the area of the curve above the diagonal line, the greater its discriminating power.
5. Range of characteristic curves make it possible to determine and then choose the appropriate cut points for the desired sensitivity or specificity.

Population Effect

1. Sensitivity and specificity are inversely related, are affected by the population tested, and are determined by the choice of a cut point or discriminate value.
2. Once a discriminate value is chosen that determines a test's specificity and sensitivity, the population tested must be considered.
3. If the population is skewed toward individuals with a

greater disease severity, the test will have a higher sensitivity. For instance, the exercise test has a higher sensitivity in individuals with triple vessel disease than in those with single vessel disease.
4. A test can have a lower specificity if it is used in individuals more likely to have false-positive test results. For instance, the exercise test has a lower specificity in individuals with mitral valve prolapse and in women.
5. The sensitivity and specificity of exercise-induced ST-segment depression can be demonstrated by analyzing the results obtained when exercise testing and coronary angiography have been used to evaluate patients. From these studies, the exercise test cut point of 0.1 mV horizontal or down-sloping ST-segment depression exhibits the following test characteristics:
   a. Specificity of 84% for angiographically significant coronary artery disease; that is, 84% of those without significant angiographic disease had normal exercise test results.
   b. Sensitivity of 66% for angiographic coronary artery disease with a range of 40% for one-vessel disease to 90% for three-vessel disease.

Relative Risk and Predictive Value

1. Two additional terms determined by sensitivity and specificity that define the diagnostic performance of a test are relative risk and predictive value. Figure 16-1 also shows how these terms are calculated. Note that both are dependent on the prevalence of disease in the population tested. Table 16-1 demonstrates how disease prevalence affects these calculations.
2. The relative risk is the relative chance of having disease if the test results are abnormal as compared with the chance of having disease if the test results are normal.
3. The predictive value of abnormal test results is the percentage of those persons with abnormal test results who have disease. Predictive value cannot be estimated directly from a test's demonstrated specificity or sensitivity but is dependent on disease prevalence, which is equivalent to pretest probability of disease.

Pretest Probability

1. The clinician's estimation of pretest probability is based on the patient's history (including age, gender, chest pain characteristics), physical examination, and

Table 16-1. Test Performance Versus Predictive Value and Risk Ratio: A Model in a Population of 10,000

Disease Prevalence	*Subjects*	*Number with Abnormal Test Results*	*Test Performance*	*Number with Normal Test Results*
5%	500 diseased	450 (TP)	90% sensitivity	50 (FN)
		350 (TP)	70% sensitivity	150 (FN)
	9500 nondiseased	2850 (FP)	70% specificity	6650 (TN)
		950 (FP)	90% specificity	8550 (TN)
50%	5000 diseased	4500 (TP)	90% sensitivity	500 (FN)
		3500 (TP)	70% sensitivity	1500 (FN)
	5000 nondiseased	1500 (FP)	70% specificity	3500 (TN)
		500 (FP)	90% specificity	4500 (TN)

	Predictive Value of Abnormal Test		*Risk Ratio**	
Disease Prevalence	5	50	5	50
Sensitivity/specificity				
70%/90%	27%	88%	27	3
90%/70%	14%	75%	14	5
90%/90%	32%	90%	64	9
66%/84%	18%	80%	9	3

TP, True-positive test result; FN, false-negative test result; FP, false-positive test result; TN, true-negative test result.
*Multiplied by that for healthy subjects.

initial testing, and the clinician's own experience with this type of problem. Table 16-2 illustrates this for middle-aged men.

2. Lack of symptoms makes the pretest probability so low that a positive test result is unlikely to be associated with disease. Screening asymptomatic populations, even those with elevated risk factors, results in misclassifying more individuals than identifying those with disease.

Table 16-2. Probability of Coronary Disease for Middle-Aged Males or Postmenopausal Females (Groups with Highest Prevalance) Before or After Any Noninvasive Test

Chest Pain Character	*Pretest*	*Postabnormal Test*	*Postnormal Test*
Typical Angina	90%	98%	75%
Atypical Angina	50%	90%	25%
Nonangina	10%	45%	4%
None	2%	6%	<1%

3. Typical angina makes the pretest probability of disease so high that the test result does not affect it much.
4. Atypical angina is a 50-50 probability, and the test result really affects the diagnostic outcome.

Probability Analysis

1. The information most important to a clinician attempting to make a diagnosis is the probability of the patient having or not having the disease once the test result is known.
2. Such a probability cannot be accurately estimated from the test result and the diagnostic characteristics of the test alone. It also requires knowledge of the probability of the patient having the disease before the test is administered (i.e., disease prevalence).
3. Bayes's theorem states that the probability of a patient having the disease after a test is performed will be the product of the disease probability before the test and the probability that the test provided a true result.
4. The clinician often makes this calculation intuitively when he suspects the abnormal test results of the exercise test of a 30-year-old woman with chest pain to be a false positive (low prior odds or probability). The same abnormal test results would be accepted as a true result in a 60-year-old man with angina who had a previous MI (high prior odds or probability).
5. Approximately 90% of the usual patients with true angina pectoris (that is, middle-aged men) have significant angiographic coronary disease. In these usual patients presenting with atypical angina pectoris, approximately 50% have been found to have significant angiographic coronary disease (see Table 16-1). Atypical angina refers to pain that has an unusual location, prolonged duration, or inconsistent precipitating factors, or that is unresponsive to nitroglycerin.

Screening

1. Screening is the application of a diagnostic test to identify disease in an apparently healthy, asymptomatic population.
2. Recent studies markedly changed the understanding of the application of exercise testing as a screening tool. These studies were additional follow-up studies and one angiographic study from the coronary artery surgery study population in which 195 individuals with abnormal exercise-induced ST depression and

normal coronary angiogram results were followed for 7 years. No increased incidence of cardiac events was found, and the concerns of increased risk have not been substantiated.

3. The new follow-up studies have had different results compared to prior studies, mainly because hard cardiac end points and not angina were required. The first ten prospective studies of exercise testing in asymptomatic individuals included angina as a cardiac disease endpoint. This led to a bias for individuals with abnormal test results to report subsequently angina or to be diagnosed as having angina. When only hard endpoints (death or MI) were used, the test could only identify a third of the patients with hard events and 95% of those with abnormal test results were false positives (did not die or have a MI). The predictive value of the abnormal exercise electrocardiogram in screening ranged from 5% to 46%, with the former being correct.
4. In the screening studies that used appropriate endpoints (and not angina pectoris), only 5% of those with abnormal test results developed coronary heart disease over the follow-up period. Thus, more than 90% of those with abnormal test results were false positives (i.e., 19 of 20 with an abnormal test result would not have a cardiac event).
5. In a Lipid Research Clinics study, only patients with elevated cholesterol were considered, and yet only a 6% positive predictive value was found.
6. Some individuals in whom coronary disease eventually develops will change on retesting from a normal to an abnormal response. However, a change from a negative to a positive test is no more predictive than is a test with initially abnormal results.
7. Thallium scintigraphy should be the first choice in evaluating asymptomatic individuals with abnormal exercise ECG results until exercise echocardiography is validated.
8. It is best to screen only those who request it, those with multiple abnormal risk factors, those with worrisome medical histories, or those with a family history of premature cardiovascular disease. It is difficult to choose a chronological age after which exercise testing is necessary as a screening technique prior to beginning an exercise program, as physiologic age is im-

portant. In general, if the exercise is more strenuous than vigorous walking, most individuals older than age 50 will benefit from such screening.

9. When the exercise test is used to classify asymptomatic individuals as having or not having coronary artery disease, it can cause harm (psychological, work and insurance status, cost for more tests, etc.) by misclassifying approximately 10% of those without coronary artery disease as having disease.
10. Rather than simply classifying the test results as abnormal or normal, it is better to use the DUKE prognostic score.

Influence of Other Factors on Test Performance

Significance and Effect of Resting ST Depression

1. Patients with resting ST-segment depression on their baseline electrocardiogram have a higher prevalence of severe coronary artery disease and a poorer long-term prognosis than patients without resting ST-segment depression.
2. Exercise-induced ST-segment depression has discriminatory power for the diagnosis of coronary artery disease in these same patients:
   a. For the diagnosis of coronary artery disease in patients without a prior MI, the criteria of 2 mm of additional exercise-induced ST-segment depression and the appearance of downward-sloping ST-segment depression during recovery, were particularly effective in these patients.
   b. For the diagnosis of severe coronary disease in patients who had survived a prior MI, the criteria of 2 mm of additional exercise-induced ST-segment depression and prolonged recovery ST-segment depression were better markers than the standard criteria.[6,7]

Alternate Criteria for Patients on Digoxin

1. Digoxin use at the time of exercise testing can lower the specificity of exercise electrocardiography as a marker for coronary artery disease.[8]
2. Persistence of exercise-induced ST-segment depression $\geq$ 4 minutes into recovery or the development of downward-sloping ST-segment depression during recovery are reasonable markers for coronary artery disease in these same patients.

Beta Blocker Therapy

1. With patients subgrouped according to Beta-blocker administration as initiated by their referring physician, no differences in test performance were found.[9]
2. For routine exercise testing in the clinical setting, it appears unnecessary for physicians to accept the risk of stopping beta blockers before testing when a patient is exhibiting possible symptoms of ischemia.

Inferior Lead ST Depression

1. Lead V_5 alone consistently outperforms the inferior leads and the combination of leads V_5 with II, because lead II had such a high false-positive rate.
2. In patients without prior MI and normal resting electrocardiogram results, precordial lead V_5 alone is a reliable marker for coronary artery disease. In addition, the monitoring of inferior limb leads adds little additional diagnostic information.
3. In patients with normal resting ECG results, exercise-induced ST-segment depression confined to the inferior leads is of little value for the identification of coronary disease.[10]

KEY POINTS IN THE DIAGNOSTIC APPLICATION OF EXERCISE TESTING

1. Evaluation of exercise testing as a diagnostic test for coronary artery disease depends on the population tested, which must be divided into those with and without coronary artery disease established by independent techniques.
2. Coronary angiography and clinical follow-up for coronary events are two methods of separating a population into those with and without coronary disease.
3. No matter what techniques are used, there is a reciprocal relationship between sensitivity and specificity. The more specific a test (i.e., the more able to determine who is disease free), the less sensitive it is and vice versa.
4. The values for sensitivity and specificity can be altered by adjusting the criterion used for abnormal. For instance, when the criterion for an abnormal exercise-induced ST-segment response is altered to 0.2-mV depression, making it more specific for coronary artery disease, the sensitivity of the test will be reduced by half.
5. For unknown reasons, the specificity of the ST-

segment response is decreased when the test is used in women and in patients who have ST-segment depression at rest, left ventricular hypertrophy, vasoregulatory abnormalities, mitral valve prolapse, and ST depression isolated to the inferior leads.

6. In studies that considered the number of coronary arteries involved, all found increasing sensitivity of the test as more vessels were involved. The greatest number of false negatives has been found among patients with single-vessel disease, particularly if the diseased vessel was not the left anterior descending artery.
7. Beta blockade does not appear to impair the accuracy of the exercise ECG.

REFERENCES

1. Guyatt GH. Readers' guide for articles evaluating diagnostic tests: What ACP Journal Club does for you and what you must do yourself. *Am Coll Phys J Club* 115:A–16, 1991.
2. Philbrick JT, Horwitz RI, Feinstein AR. Methodologic problems of exercise testing for coronary artery disease: Groups, analysis and bias. *Am J Cardiol* 46:807, 1980.
3. Rosanski A, Diamond GA, Berman DS, Forrester JS, Morris D, Swan HJ. The declining specificity of exercise radionuclide ventriculography. *N Engl J Med* 309:518–522, 1983.
4. Detrano R, Yiannikas J, Salcedo EE, Rincon G, Go RT, Williams G, Leatherman J. Bayesian probability analysis: A prospective demonstration of its clinical utility in diagnosing coronary disease. *Circulation* 69:541–550, 1984.
5. Gianrossi R, Detrano R, Mulvihill D, Lehmann K, Dubach P, Colombo A, McArthur D, Froelicher VF. Exercise-induced ST depression in the diagnosis of coronary artery disease: A meta-analysis. *Circulation* 80:87–98, 1989.
6. Detrano R, Gianrossi R, Froelicher VF. The diagnostic accuracy of the exercise electrocardiogram: A meta-analysis of 22 years of research. *Prog Cardiovasc Dis* 33:173–205, 1989.
7. Callaham PR, Thomas L, Ellestad MH. Prolonged ST-segment depression following exercise predicts significant proximal left coronary artery stenosis. *Circulation* 76(suppl IV):IV–253, 1987.
8. Sundqvist K, Atterhog JH, Jogestrand T. Effect of di-

goxin on the electrocardiogram at rest and during exercise in healthy subjects. *Am J Cardiol* 57:661–665, 1986.

9. Herbert WG, Dubach P, Lehmann KG, Froelicher VF. Effect of beta-blockade on the interpretation of the exercise ECG: ST level versus ST/HR index. *Am Heart J* 122:993–1000, 1991.
10. Miranda CP, Liu J, Kadar A, Janosi A, Froning J, Lehmann KG, Froelicher VF. Usefulness of exercise-induced ST-segment depression in the inferior leads during exercise testing as a marker for coronary artery disease. *Am J Cardiol* 69:303–308, 1992.

Prognostic Applications

There are two principal reasons for estimating prognosis:

1. To provide accurate answers to patient's questions regarding the probable outcome of their illness.
2. To identify those patients in whom interventions might improve outcome.

Clinical features are extremely important for pretest stratification. Ischemic signs/symptoms alone are associated with a 2% annual cardiac mortality, whereas congestive heart failure signs/symptoms alone or in combination with ischemia are associated with a 25% annual cardiac mortality. In addition, patients in the first 3 months after a myocardial infarction (MI) are exposed to a 10% mortality risk.

PATHOPHYSIOLOGIC PRINCIPLES

The basic pathophysiologic features of coronary artery disease that determine prognosis include:

Arrhythmic risk
Amount of remaining myocardium (reflected by left ventricular (LV) function)
Amount of myocardium in jeopardy

Arrhythmic risk does not appear to be independently predicted by exercise testing as the prognosis for arrhythmias is closely related to left ventricular abnormalities.

RESPONSES WITH PROGNOSTIC SIGNIFICANCE

Ischemic Responses

The exercise responses due to ischemia include the following:

Angina
ST-segment depression
ST-segment elevation over ECG areas without Q-waves

Responses Due to Either or Both Ischemia and Left Ventricular Dysfunction

The responses due either to ischemia or LV dysfunction include the following:

Chronotropic incompetence or heart rate impairment
Systolic blood pressure abnormalities[1] (exercise-induced hypotension)
Poor exercise capacity

The association of ischemia and LV dysfunction explains why they are so important in predicting prognosis.

1. Exercise-induced dysrhythmias indicate electrical instability most often due to LV dysfunction rather than ischemia (except for ST elevation in a normal ECG, which is very arrythmogenic) and do not appear to have independent predictive power.
2. The only response specifically associated with LV dysfunction is ST elevation over diagnostic Q-waves (i.e., post-MI). This carries an increased risk in these patients and indicates that they have depressed LV function and possibly larger aneurysms compared with those with Q-waves without elevation.
3. Exercise capacity poorly correlates with LV function (even in patients without signs or symptoms of right-sided heart failure).[2] Right-sided failure usually worsens any limitations.
4. Exercise testing is not very helpful in identifying patients with moderate LV dysfunction, an important marker for improved survival with bypass surgery. This is better recognized by a history of congestive heart failure (CHF), physical examination, resting ECG, echocardiogram, or radionuclide ventriculography.

STABLE CORONARY ARTERY DISEASE

Rationale for Deciding Who Needs to See a Cardiologist

1. When **symptoms (specifically angina)** cannot be controlled by medications, catheterization is indicated. However, in issues involving prolongation of life, decisions are more problematic.
2. Although angiographic surrogates can be used (severe coronary artery disease [CAD]), it is preferable to rely on follow-up studies. These studies are difficult and expensive and, when completed, require special statistical methods called survival analysis for analysis.

Predicting Coronary Angiographic Results

Meta-analysis Predicting Severity of Angiographic Disease

To evaluate the variability in the reported accuracy of the exercise ECG for predicting severe coronary disease, a meta-analysis was performed on 60 reports comparing exercise-induced ST depression with coronary angiographic findings.[3] The 60 reports included 12,030 patients who underwent both tests. Three variables were found to be related to sensitivity: the exclusion of patients with right bundle branch block, the comparison with another exercise test believed to be superior in accuracy, and the exclusion of patients taking digitalis (mean sensitivity 86%; mean specificity 53% for left main or triple vessel disease). A similar analysis[4] found that the 1-mm criterion averaged a sensitivity of 75% and a specificity of 66%, whereas the 2-mm criterion averaged a sensitivity of 52% and a specificity of 86%. From these two reviews, it is obvious that the exercise ECG has excellent characteristics for identifying patients with severe angiographic disease.

Angiographic Studies of Silent Ischemia

In a review of the angiographic studies of silent ischemia[5] encompassing almost 6,000 patients, a consistent finding was that patients with symptomatic ischemia had a higher prevalence of severe angiographic disease than did patients with silent ischemia.

Predicting Cardiac Endpoints

Survival Analysis

1. The most reliable prediction endpoint is cardiovascular death. Studies that include coronary artery bypass surgery (CABS) as an endpoint are not valid because the test results are used to decide who undergoes these procedures.
2. The two most commonly used survival techniques are Kaplan-Meier survival curves for univariate analysis and the Cox Hazzard model for multivariate analysis.
3. Multivariate analysis is necessary because many of the variables interact.
4. Univariately, variables can be associated with death, but the association may be through other variables. For instance, digoxin use is associated with death through CHF, whereas exercise-induced ST elevation associates with death through the underlying Q-waves.

Results of Correctly Performed Studies

1. Of the nine studies of patients with stable coronary disease that used multivariate survival analysis techniques to predict prognosis, two appropriately pre-

dicted time to cardiovascular death using a score formed by the variables chosen and their relative weights.[6,7]

2. Exercise-induced ST depression can be falsely excluded from predictive models because of work-up bias.
3. The VAMC prognostic score can estimate the average annual cardiovascular mortality in male veterans being evaluated for stable coronary artery disease, obviating the need for cardiac catheterization in many of these patients.
4. The Duke score is recommended in the general population, particularly when women are included.
5. These important prognostic scores and their components are listed in Fig. 17-1.

Use of the Duke Nomogram

A nomogram that facilitates application of the Duke score is Fig. 17-2. Use of this nomogram permits an estimate of a patient's mortality from cardiovascular disease, which can be compared with that expected from age, gender, and race (based on the National Center for Health Statistics) and to the mortality expected from bypass surgery based on the Parsonnet case mix score. It is important to note that the nomogram probably underestimates prognosis in patients with CHF and is not valid within 6 months of an MI.

Prognostic Studies of Silent Ischemia during Exercise Testing

Preliminary studies led to the hypothesis that "silent" myocardial ischemia had a worse prognosis than angina pectoris because patients with it do not have an intact "warning system." However, in studies of patients referred for diagnostic purposes or with stable coronary syndromes, silent myocardial ischemia detected by exercise testing has been associated with either a lesser or similar

Fig. 17-1. The Duke University and Veterans Affairs prognostic scores and their components. AP, angina pectoris; dig, digoxin; CHF, congestive heart failure; E-I, exercise induced; SBP, systolic blood pressure; TM, treadmill.

Duke score = METs − 5 × (mm E-I ST depression) − 4 × (TM AP index)
VA score = 5 × (CHF/dig) + mm E-I ST depression + Change in SBP score − METs
Treadmill angina pectoris (TM AP): 0 if no angina, 1 if angina occurred during test, 2 if angina was the reason for stopping
CHF/dig score: 0 if no history of CHF and patient not receiving digoxin, if history of CHF or patient receiving digoxin
Change in SBP score: from 0 for rise greater than 40 mm Hg to 5 for drop below rest (scored in increments of 10 mm Hg)

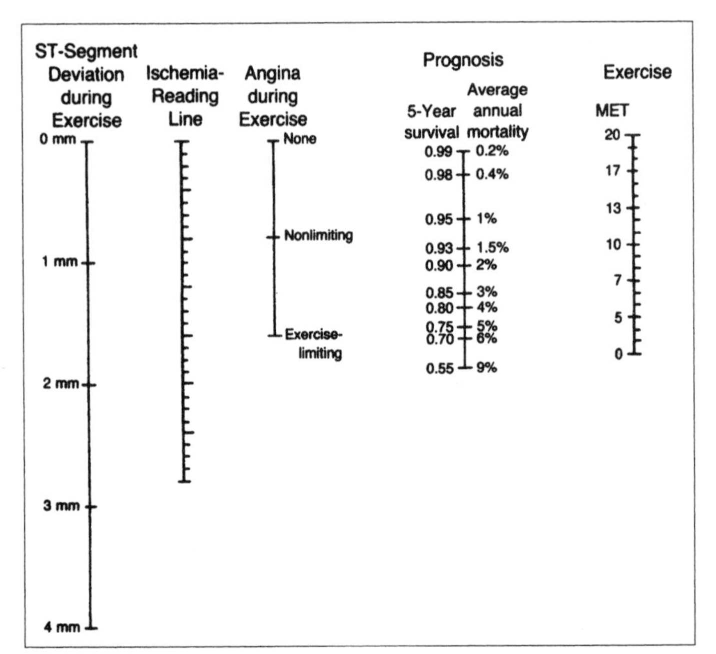

Fig. 17-2. The nomogram for the Duke University prognostic score based on the equation listed in Figure 17-1. Mark the amount of ST depression and angina score. Connect the points between the ST depression mark and the angina score to determine the point on the ischemia reading line. Last, connect the point on the ischemia reading scale with METS achieved. The point marked on the prognosis scale estimates mortality.

prognosis for these patients compared with patients with angina pectoris.[8]

Key Points of Prognostication in Stable Coronary Artery Disease

1. There is much information supporting the use of exercise testing as the first noninvasive step after the history, physical examination, and resting ECG in the prognostic evaluation of coronary artery disease patients.
2. It accomplishes both purposes of prognostic testing: It provides information regarding the patient's status and helps make recommendations for optimal management.
3. The exercise test results help the physician to make reasonable decisions for selection of patients who should undergo coronary angiography. Simple clinical and exercise test scores can be used to decide which

patients need interventions to improve their prognosis; these scores frequently obviate the need for cardiac catheterization.

4. The VAMC score is recommended for the male veteran population and the Duke score for the general population, including women.
5. Patients can be given estimates of their relative annual mortality with medical versus surgical therapy using scores and case mix data.[9]
6. Quality of life issues cannot be resolved with such scores; these issues require an understanding physician and an informed patient.
7. In general, physicians overestimate the danger of ischemia; perhaps if physicians were given accurate mortality estimates, the practice of medicine would be more conservative.

POSTMYOCARDIAL INFARCTION EXERCISE TESTING

Safety of Exercise Testing Early After Myocardial Infarction

The risk of death and major arrhythmias from performing an exercise test soon after MI is very small. However, the major research is based on clinically selected MI patients: those without major complications such as heart failure, severe arrhythmias, or ischemia. The risk is highest in those rejected for testing for these clinical reasons. The exercise test can determine the possible risk the patient may incur with exercise, and it is certainly safer that adverse reactions be observed in controlled circumstances.

Characteristics that lead to the classification of an MI as complicated with an associated higher mortality or poor prognosis include the following:

CHF
Cardiogenic shock
Large MI as determined by creatinine phosphokinase or ECG
Pericarditis
Dangerous arrhythmias including conduction problems
Concurrent illnesses
Pulmonary embolus
Continued ischemia
Stroke or transient ischemic attack

Exercise testing in these patients should be delayed or omitted from their evaluation because of the high risk.

Some patients must go directly to cardiac catheterization or undergo a nonexercise stress procedure.

When to Perform an Exercise Test

The post-MI exercise test can be performed just prior to discharge from the hospital or after discharge, usually within 3 months or whenever the patient is ready to return to full activities. Because there are benefits specific to both timings, most patients should be tested at both intervals.

Predischarge Testing

Submitting patients to exercise testing can expedite and optimize their discharge from the hospital and has been performed as early as 3 days after an MI. The patient's response to exercise, work capacity, and limiting factors at the time of discharge can be assessed by the exercise test. A patient should not get the impression that if he or she "fails" the test he will end up in the cardiac catheterization laboratory.

An exercise test prior to discharge is important for giving a patient guidelines for exercise at home, reassuring him or her regarding physical status, and determining the risk of complications. The benefits of a test at this time include the following:

Setting safe exercise levels (exercise prescription).
Optimizing discharge.
Altering medical therapy.
Triaging for intensity of follow-up.
First step in rehabilitation (assurance, encouragement).
Reassuring a spouse or significant other.
Recognizing exercise-induced ischemia and dysrhythmias.

SAFETY LIMITS

1. Heart rate limit of 140 beats/min and a MET level of 7 is used for patients younger than 40, and 130 beats/min and a MET level of 5 for patients older than 40.
2. Particularly for patients on beta blockers, a Borg perceived exertion level in the range of 16 is used to end the test.
3. Conservative clinical indications for stopping the test should be applied.

Postdischarge Testing

Another test 3 weeks or longer later provides a safe basis for advising the patient to resume or increase his or her activity level and return to work. Patient and spouse confidence can be enhanced by the test also.[10] The benefits of a test at this time include the following:

Determining limitations
Reassuring employers
Determining level of disability
Triaging for invasive studies
Deciding on medications
Prescribing exercise
Continuing rehabilitation

Rationale for Determining Who Should See the Cardiologist

This is easy to decide when **symptoms (specifically angina)** cannot be controlled, but otherwise it is often difficult to decide who should be considered for intervention to prolong life. To answer this question, studies using angiographic surrogates (severe CAD) and follow-up studies must be considered.

Predicting Coronary Angiographic Results

1. For exercise testing results to be clinically helpful in deciding about CABS, the exercise test must predict which patients have anatomic findings associated with improved survival if CABS is performed: that is, left main or triple vessel disease accompanied by an ejection fraction (EF) of 30% to 50%.
2. The angiographic studies indicate that exercise testing has an average sensitivity for severe angiographic disease of 58% and an average specificity of 82%.[11,12]
3. Thus, the exercise test can identify patients with much muscle in jeopardy due to lesions causing ischemia, but it cannot recognize individuals with decreased ventricular function. Such patients are best recognized by a combination of prior history of MI or CHF, an abnormal ECG, and physical examination and chest radiographic findings.

Predicting Cardiac Endpoints

The 28 studies using exercise testing in the early post-MI period, with a follow-up for cardiac events, have been subjected to metaanalysis.[13] The five exercise test variables suggested to have prognostic importance are as follows:

1. ST-segment depression (and sometimes elevation).

2. Exercise test-induced angina.
3. Poor exercise capacity or excessive heart rate response to a low workload.
4. Blunted systolic blood pressure (SBP) response (or exertional hypotension).
5. Premature ventricular contractions.

Only SBP and exercise capacity have a greater than chance predictive value in these 28 studies. ST depression with exercise effectively identifies high risk only in patients after a non-Q-wave MI.[14,15] The difference in the prognostic value of the post-MI exercise ECG between studies is due to variations in the prevalence of Q-wave versus non-Q-wave MI among study populations.

Who Needs Coronary Artery Bypass Surgery After Myocardial Infarction?

1. By considering known associations and relationships, the clinical description of the high-risk patient who could potentially have improved survival with CABS can be derived.
2. The randomized trials of CABS have demonstrated that patients with triple-vessel or left main disease with an EF of 30% to 50% have improved survival with surgery compared with medical therapy.
3. The clinical picture, either by history or by ECG, that would result in an EF from 30% to 50% would include patients with large anterior MI, a history or ECG pattern of multiple MI, transmural MI followed by subendocardial MI, or a history of transient congestive heart failure with an MI. In addition, physical findings of ventricular dyskinesia or cardiomegaly on palpation would support this.
4. Thus, clinical and electrocardiographic features predict those with decreased ventricular function.
5. Noninvasive testing (i.e., radionuclide ventriculography and echocardiography) could also be used to evaluate LV function.
6. Although its sensitivity is decreased in one- or two-vessel disease, the exercise ECG is approximately 90% sensitive for triple-vessel or left main disease. Angina is also very common in this group of patients.
7. Therefore, the following profile identifies the high-risk patient after an MI who should undergo coronary angiography: the patient with a history consistent with a large amount of damage (multiple MIs, abnormal pre-

cordial movements, or a history of transient congestive heart failure) or ECG findings of a large anterior MI and signs and symptoms of severe myocardial ischemia on the exercise test. Severe ischemia is characterized by the occurrence of ST-segment depression, angina, or both at a double product less than 20,000 and at less than 5 METS exercise capacity.

8. If there are no contraindications to CABS in these patients, they should be considered for coronary angiography. Post-MI patients who should be considered for reasons other than improved survival are those in whom angina is not controlled satisfactorily with medications and those in whom either the diagnosis of MI or the cause of chest pain post-MI is uncertain.

Key Points of Postmyocardial Infarction Exercise Testing

1. The test can demonstrate to the patient, relatives, or employer the effect of the MI on the capacity for physical performance.
2. Psychologically, it can cause an improvement in the patient's self-confidence by making the patient less anxious about daily physical activities.
3. The test has been helpful in reassuring spouses of post-MI patients of their physical capabilities.
4. The psychological effect of performing well on the exercise test is impressive. Many patients increase their activity and actually rehabilitate themselves after being encouraged and reassured by their response to this test.
5. A consistent finding in the review of the post-MI exercise test studies reveals that patients referred for exercise testing were at lower risk than patients not tested. This finding supports the clinical judgment of the skilled clinician for identifying high-risk patients.
6. An abnormal SBP response or a low exercise capacity were the only variables associated with a poor outcome in the meta-analysis. These responses are very powerful because they are associated with either ischemic or CHF cardiovascular deaths.
7. In the non-Q-wave MI patient, exercise-induced ST depression predicts a poor outcome and increased risk.

REFERENCES

1. Dubach P, Froelicher VF, Klein J, Oakes D, Grover-McKay M. Exercise-induced hypotension in a veteran

population: Criteria, causes, and prognosis. *Circulation* 78:1380–1387, 1988.
2. McKirnan MD, Sullivan M, Jensen D, Froelicher VF. Treadmill performance and cardiac function in selected patients with coronary heart disease. *J Am Coll Cardiol* 3:253–261, 1984.
3. Detrano R, Gianrossi R, Mulvihill D, Lehmann K, Dubach P, Colombo A, Froelicher VF. Exercise-induced ST segment depression in the diagnosis of multivessel coronary disease: A meta analysis. *J Am Coll Cardiol* 14:1501–1508, 1989.
4. Hartz A, Gammaitoni C, Young M. Quantitative analysis of the exercise tolerance test for determining the severity of coronary artery disease. *Int J Cardiol* 24:63–71, 1989.
5. Miranda C, Lehmann K, Lachterman B, Coodley G, Froelicher V. Comparison of silent and symptomatic ischemia during exercise testing in men. *Ann Intern Med* 114:649–656, 1991.
6. Mark DB, Hlatky MA, Harrell FE, Lee KL, Califf RM, Pryor DB. Exercise treadmill score for predicting prognosis in coronary artery disease. *Ann Intern Med* 106:793–800, 1987.
7. Morrow K, Morris C, Froelicher V, Thomas R, Lehmann K. The prognostic value of the exercise test in a male veteran population. *Ann Intern Med* 118:689–695, 1992.
8. Mark DB, Hlatky MA, Califf RM, Morris JJ, Sisson SD, McCants CB, Lee KL, Harrell FE, Pryor DB. Painless exercise ST deviation on the treadmill: Long-term prognosis. *J Am Coll Cardiol* 14:885–892, 1989.
9. Parsonnet V, Dean D, Bernstein A. A method of uniform stratification of risk for evaluating the results in acquired adult heart disease. *Circulation* 79(suppl I):1-3–1-12, 1989.
10. Ewart CK, Taylor CB, Reese LB, DeBusk RF. Effects of early postmyocardial infarction exercise testing on self-perception and subsequent physical activity. *Am J Cardiol* 51:1076–1080, 1983.
11. De Feyter PJ, van den Brand M, Serruys PW, Wijns W. Early angiography after myocardial infarction: What have we learned? *Am Heart J* 109:194–199, 1985.
12. Laupacis A, LaBelle R, Goeree R, Cairns J. The cost-effectiveness of routine post myocardial infarction exercise stress testing. *Can J Cardiol* 6:157–163, 1990.

13. Froelicher V, Risch M, Perdue S, Pewen W. Meta-Analysis of the studies of exercise testing after MI. *Am J Med* 6:769–772, 1987.
14. Klein J, Froelicher V, Detrano R. Does the Rest ECG after MI determine the predictive value of exercise-induced ST depression? *J Am Coll Cardiol* 14:305–311, 1989.
15. Krone R, Dwyer E, Greenberg H. Risk stratification in patients with first non-Q wave MI: The Multicenter Post-MI Research Group. *J Am Coll Cardiol* 14:31–37, 1989.

Other Applications

EVALUATION OF EXERCISE CAPACITY

Exercise testing is also performed to evaluate a patient's exercise capacity. The information obtained can allow the health care provider to institute or reevaluate an exercise prescription.

1. No questionnaire or submaximal test or nonexercise stress test can give the same results as a symptom-limited exercise test.
2. Surgical patients recovering from congenital heart defect repair, valvular replacement, and cardiac transplant can be referred for exercise capacity evaluation.
3. Other chronically ill groups evaluated for exercise capacity include patients with congestive heart failure (CHF), diabetes, chronic renal failure, and pulmonary disease.

Congestive Heart Failure

Exercise testing currently is often performed in patients with CHF for the following reasons:

1. Although it remains controversial, some studies have suggested that prognosis can be estimated by exercise capacity.
2. Because the importance of an exercise program has recently been emphasized in CHF patients, an exercise test is performed to develop an exercise prescription and monitor its progress. This can be as simple as determining a safe level of exercise and then recommending that it be performed for at least 30 minutes a day.
3. Cardiac transplantation is usually reserved for eligible patients only if their measured Vo_2 maximum is less than 6 METS.
4. The response of exercise capacity to therapies can be documented by serial exercise testing.

Disability Evaluation

Because it can objectively demonstrate exercise capacity, exercise testing is used for disability evaluation rather than relying on functional classifications.

1. Disabilities can be clarified with exercise testing and can be monitored through serial testing.
2. The MET level obtained can be related to symptoms,

usual and job-related activities, and expectations for matched age and gender.

MET levels have been established for most activities, including jobs. Even the cardiac response to isometric work can be estimated from the treadmill test.

EVALUATION OF TREATMENTS

The exercise test can be used to evaluate the effects of both medical and surgical treatment. The effects of various medications including nitrates, digitalis, antiarrhythmics, and antihypertensive agents have been evaluated by exercise testing.

One problem with using treadmill time or workload rather than maximal oxygen uptake measurements in serial studies is that people learn to perform treadmill walking. Consequently, treadmill time or workload, frequently used in drug studies, increases during serial studies without any improvement in cardiovascular function (i.e., VO_2 max or cardiac output). Measurement of ventilatory oxygen uptake can avoid the problem of learning, making it advantageous when the effects of medical or surgical treatment are being evaluated by treadmill testing.

Medications

Antianginal Agents

Antianginal drug studies look for an increase in exercise capacity, loss of angina, and increased double product before angina, ST depression, or both occur.

The reproducibility of exercise testing[1] and safety of placebo in studying antianginal agents have been studied. When all events leading to dropout from trials of 12 antianginal drugs submitted in support of new drug applications to the Food and Drug Administration were followed,[2] there were few adverse experiences associated with short-term placebo use. Withholding active treatment for angina does not increase the risk of serious cardiac events.

Congestive Heart Failure

1. Digoxin and angiotensin-converting enzyme inhibitors have been studied and appear to increase exercise capacity in heart failure patients.
2. Although exercise capacity has been improved by certain medications, survival has not always been similarly benefited.

3. With vasodilators, the blood pressure response can be considerably blunted.

Antihypertensive Agents
These agents have been studied particularly for those patients who experience hypertension during exercise.

Surgical Interventions

1. Exercise testing has been used to evaluate patients before and after coronary artery bypass surgery (CABS), coronary angioplasty, and cardiac transplantation.
2. The studies of CABS and percutaneous transluminal coronary angioplasty (PTCA) are confounded by differences in medications before and after intervention. In addition, there is a low rate of abnormal preintervention studies in the patients undergoing PTCA, who mostly have single-vessel disease.
3. Although preprocedural documentation of ischemia is indicated prior to PTCA, prediction of restenosis using the exercise test has not been possible.[3]

MISCELLANEOUS APPLICATIONS

Evaluation of Patients for Noncardiac Surgery
The exercise test has not been justified as a routine means of evaluating patients prior to surgery as a replacement or even an addition to the Goldman or Detsky indices.[4] However, it is frequently requested by anesthesiologists who prefer to alter their approaches if the patient is known to have ischemia.

Evaluation of Dysrhythmias
An exercise test can be used to evaluate patients with dysrhythmias or to induce dysrhythmias in patients with the appropriate exercise-related symptoms.

1. The dysrhythmias that can be evaluated include premature ventricular contractions (PVC), sick sinus syndrome, and various degrees of heart block.
2. Maximal exercise testing can be useful for detection of arrhythmias and assessment of antiarrhythmic drug efficacy.[5]
3. Maximal exercise testing can be conducted safely in patients with malignant arrhythmias. Clinical variables previously considered to confer risk during exercise are not predictive of complications.

Evaluation of Valvular Heart Disease

Exercise testing has been used in the evaluation of patients with valvular heart disease.

1. It has been used to qualify the amount of disability caused by the disease, to reproduce any exercise-induced symptomatology, and to evaluate the patient's response to medical and surgical intervention.
2. The exercise ECG has been used as a means to identify concurrent coronary artery disease (CAD), but there is a high prevalence of false-positive responses (ST depression not due to ischemia) because of the frequent baseline ECG abnormalities and left ventricular (LV) hypertrophy.
3. Some physicians have used the exercise test to help decide when surgery is indicated.

Aortic Stenosis

Exercise testing has been used most in patients with aortic stenosis (AS).[6,7]

1. Effort syncope in patients with aortic stenosis occurs and is a symptom of significant obstruction.
2. Most guidelines regarding exercise testing list moderate to severe aortic stenosis as a contraindication for exercise testing due to concern with syncope and cardiac arrest.
3. Guidelines for monitoring patients with aortic stenosis during exercise testing, and clinical situations in which exercise testing must be performed, include frequent blood pressure measurement (usually every 1–2 minutes) and a conservative tendency to terminate. Usually, echocardiography is indicated prior to an exercise test in patients with a significant systolic murmur to estimate the degree of stenosis.
4. Systolic blood pressure should be followed very closely in these patients (every minute and with any change in signs or symptoms).
5. Exercise plays an important role in the objective assessment of symptoms, hemodynamic response, and functional capacity, even in patients with aortic stenosis.
6. Whether ST-segment depression indicates significant CAD or not remains unclear; it could be due to inadequate cardiac output and cardiac hypertrophy.
7. By performing exercise testing preoperatively and

postoperatively, the exercise capacity benefits of surgery and baseline impairment can be quantified.

8. Exercise testing offers the opportunity to evaluate objectively any disparities between history and clinical findings, for example, in the elderly "asymptomatic subject" with physical or Doppler findings of severe aortic stenosis.
9. Often the echocardiographic studies are inadequate in such patients, particularly when they are smokers.
10. When Doppler echocardiography reveals a significant gradient in the asymptomatic patient with normal exercise capacity, he or she should be followed up closely until symptoms develop.
11. In patients with an inadequate systolic blood pressure response to exercise or a fall in systolic blood pressure from the resting value when symptoms occur, surgery appears to be indicated.

REFERENCES

1. Sullivan M, Genter F, Savvides M, Roberts M, Myers J, Froelicher V. The reproducibility of hemodynamic, electrocardiographic, and gas exchange data during treadmill exercise in patients with stable angina pectoris. *Chest* 86:375–382, 1984.
2. Glasser SP, Clark PI, Lipicky RJ, Hubbard JM, Yusuf S. Exposing patients with chronic, stable, exertional angina to placebo periods in drug trials. *JAMA* 265: 1550–1554, 1991.
3. Honan MB, Bengtson JR, Pryor DB, Rendall DS, Stack RS, Hinohara T, Skelton TN, Califf RM, Hlatky MA, Mark DB. Exercise treadmill testing is a poor predictor of anatomic restenosis after angioplasty for acute myocardial infarction. *Circulation* 80:1585–1594, 1989.
4. Carliner NH, Fisher ML, Plotnick GD, Garbart H, Rapoport A, Kelemen MH, Moran GW. Routine preoperative exercise testing in patients undergoing major noncardiac surgery. *Am J Cardiol* 56:51–58, 1985.
5. Young DZ, Lampert S, Graboys TB, Lown B. Safety of maximal exercise testing in patients at high risk for ventricular arrhythmia. *Circulation* 70:184–191, 1984.
6. Areskog NH. Exercise testing in the evaluation of patients with valvular aortic stenosis. *Clin Physiol* 4: 201–208, 1984.
7. Atwood JE, Kawanishi S, Myers J, Froelicher VF. Exercise and the heart: Exercise testing in patients with aortic stenosis. *Chest* 93:1083–1087, 1988.

Key Points from Part IV

The exercise test can be used to evaluate the effects of both medical and surgical treatment. For example, the effects of various medications, including antianginal, digitalis, antiarrhythmic, and antihypertensive agents, can be evaluated with exercise testing.

The studies evaluating antianginal agents have been greatly hampered by the increase in treadmill time that occurs merely by performing serial tests. For this reason, expired gas analysis is frequently added to protocols evaluating therapeutic agents.

Patients with congestive heart failure, angina, or valvular heart disease, alone or in combination, can be assessed.

Considerable care must be taken when administering exercise testing to patients with aortic stenosis. Blood pressures should be taken often and the test stopped if systolic blood pressure drops. When the severity of the stenosis is uncertain, an echocardiogram should be performed prior to testing.

Exercise testing is also performed to evaluate a patient's exercise capacity, and the information obtained can allow the health care provider to institute or reevaluate an exercise prescription.

Disabilities can be clarified with exercise testing and can be monitored through serial testing. Because it can objectively demonstrate exercise capacity, exercise testing is used for disability evaluation rather than relying on functional classifications.

The studies of coronary artery bypass surgery and percutaneous transluminal coronary angioplasty (PTCA) are confounded by differences in medications before and after intervention and by the low rate of abnormal preintervention studies in the patients undergoing PTCA who mostly have single-vessel disease. Standard exercise testing does not appear to be very helpful in predicting restenosis.

The results from studies determining the risk of exercise-induced premature ventricular contractions and more serious ventricular dysrhythmias are mixed, but prognosis appears to relate more to any coexisting conditions than to the arrhythmias themselves. Some investigators contend that exercise testing is a better means of evaluating patients with problematic arrhythmias than other testing modalities. Certainly, exercise-induced arrhythmias are best studied with exercise.

Worksheet for Exercise Testing

I. Preliminary Patient Preparation

[ ] 1. Consent signed (less than 1 in 10,000 event rate; less for death)
[ ] 2. SAQ Questionnaire completed
[ ] 3. No food intake or smoking for 3 hours

II. Patient Interview: Ask specific questions regarding the following and review records.

[ ] 1. Past medical history (with dates)

A. Cardiovascular

[ ] CHF
[ ] MI
[ ] PVD
[ ] HTN
[ ] PTCA
[ ] Stroke
[ ] Congenital
[ ] Syncope
[ ] Arrhythmia
[ ] Pacemaker
[ ] Sudden death
[ ] Valve disease
[ ] Cardiac catheter
[ ] Atrial fibrillation

B. Cardiovascular Surgery

[ ] CABG
[ ] Carotid
[ ] Aorto femoral
[ ] AoV replacement
[ ] Mitral V repair
[ ] Mitral V replacement

C. Other medical disease

[ ] Diabetes mellitus
[ ] Musculoskeletal disease
[ ] Cancer
[ ] COPD
[ ] Anemia
[ ] Thyroid disease

[ ] 2. Family History

[ ] Family history (CAD in blood relative < 65 years)
[ ] Heart muscle disease
[ ] Sudden death

[ ] 3. Risk Factors

[ ] HTN
[ ] DM
[ ] Sedentary
[ ] Obesity
[ ] Tobacco smoking
[ ] Cholesterol

[ ] 4. Current Symptoms

[ ] PND
[ ] Orthopnea
[ ] Edema
[ ] Weight change
[ ] Palpitation
[ ] Angina
[ ] Wheezing
[ ] LOC/syncope
[ ] Claudication
[ ] GI symptoms
[ ] Neurological symptom
[ ] Noncardiac chest pain

[ ] 5. Chest Pain History

[ ] Typical angina
[ ] Atypical angina
[ ] Noncardiac chest pain
[ ] Variant angina
[ ] Unstable angina
[ ] None

[ ] 6. Medication Review

[ ] Digoxin
[ ] Ca+Antag
[ ] ASA
[ ] ACE
[ ] Anti-HTN
[ ] Nitrates
[ ] Coumadin
[ ] Insulin
[ ] Beta-blocker
[ ] Antiarrhythmic
[ ] Diuretics
[ ] Lipid agent

[ ] 7. Activity Status

[ ] Review SAQ questionnaire
[ ] Previous treadmill experience and complications
[ ] Complications with activity

III. Patient Examination

[ ] 1. Vital Signs—Heart Rate, BP (BP Controlled)

[ ] 2. Cardiovascular Examination

[ ] JVP
[ ] Carotid
[ ] Heart (R/O Aortic Stenosis)
[ ] Systolic murmur
[ ] Cardiomegaly

[ ] 3. Pulmonary

[ ] 4. Periphery

[ ] Peripheral pulses
[ ] Edema
[ ] Carotid bruits
[ ] Femoral bruits

5. Musculoskeletal

[ ] Gait assessment

IV. Reason for Exercise Test

1. [ ] Diagnosis
[ ] Prognosis
[ ] Exercise capacity
[ ] Treatment assessment

2. [ ] Pretest probability determined

V. Data Review

[ ] Review medical chart
[ ] Review PFT
[ ] Review previous tests

[ ] ETT
[ ] Echo
[ ] Cath
[ ] MUGA
[ ] Holter
[ ] Perfusion scan

[ ] Compare Serial ECG

[ ] Prior ECG
[ ] Baseline supine ECG
[ ] Baseline standing ECG
[ ] LBBB
[ ] RBBB
[ ] WPW
[ ] LVH
[ ] ST depression

VI. Equipment Check

[ ] Estimate METS, enter target
[ ] Check ECG leads/tracing for artifact
[ ] Check emergency equipment

VII. Patient Instruction

[ ] Chest pain scale
[ ] Borg scale
[ ] Explain procedure during testing (frequent BP, symptom assessment)
[ ] Explain getting on and off of the treadmill
[ ] Demo walk

ACE, angiotensin-converting enzyme; ASA, acetylsalicylic acid; CABG, coronary artery bypass graft; CAD, coronary artery disease; CHF, congestive heart failure; COPD, chronic obstructive pulmonary disease; DM, diastolic murmur; ETT, exercise tolerance test; HTN, hypertension; JVP, jugular venous pulse; LBBB, left bundle branch block; LOC, loss of consciousness; LVH, left ventricular hypertrophy; MI, myocardial infarction; MUGA, multi-gated acquisition; PFT, pulmonary function test; PND, paroxysmal nocturnal dyspnea; PTCA, percutaneous transluminal coronary angioplasty; PVD, peripheral vascular disease; RBBB, right bundle branch block; SAQ, specific activity questionnaire; WPW, Wolff-Parkinson-White.

Index

Note: Page numbers followed by *f* indicate figures; those followed by *t* indicate tables.